Engage the Group
Engage the Brain

Engage the Group
Engage the Brain

100 Experiential Activities for Addiction Treatment

KAY COLBERT
ROXANNA ERICKSON-KLEIN

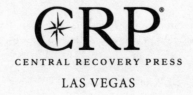

CENTRAL RECOVERY PRESS

LAS VEGAS

Central Recovery Press (CRP) is committed to publishing exceptional materials addressing addiction treatment, recovery, and behavioral healthcare topics, including original and quality books, audio/visual communications, and web-based new media. Through a diverse selection of titles, we seek to contribute a broad range of unique resources for professionals, recovering individuals and their families, and the general public.

For more information, visit www.centralrecoverypress.com.

Publisher: Central Recovery Press
          3321 N. Buffalo Drive
          Las Vegas, NV 89129

20 19 18 17 16 15   1 2 3 4 5

ISBN: 978-1-937612-89-4 (paper)
       978-1-937612-90-0 (e-book)

Photos of Kay Colbert and Roxanna Erickson-Klein used with permission.

LIMITED PHOTOCOPY LICENSE

Grateful acknowledgment is made to reprint the following:
The AA Twelve Steps are reprinted with permission of Alcoholics Anonymous World Services, Inc.

The NA Twelve Steps are reprinted by permission of NA World Services, Inc.

All quotations used with individual permission or permission from the estate of:
Rubin Battino, Milton H. Erickson, Patrick Carnes, Pennie Johnson Carnes, Kristina Erickson, Stephen Gilligan, and Ernest Rossi.

Publisher's Note: This book contains general information about addiction, addiction recovery, and related matters. The information is not medical advice, and should not be treated as such. Central Recovery Press makes no representations or warranties in relation to the information in this book. If you have any specific questions about any medical matter discussed in this book, you should consult your doctor or other professional healthcare provider. This book is not an alternative to medical advice from your doctor or other professional healthcare provider.

Our books represent the experiences and opinions of their authors only. Every effort has been made to ensure that events, institutions, and statistics presented in our books as facts are accurate and up-to-date.

Cover design by David Hardy
Interior design and layout by Deb Tremper, Six Penny Graphics

To the men, women, and children
who struggle with addiction

Contents

Foreword

This highly innovative volume, *Engage the Group, Engage the Brain: 100 Experiential Activities for Addiction Treatment* by Kay Colbert and Roxanna Erickson-Klein, brings a refreshingly new neuroscience approach to psychotherapy. It embraces a long tradition for facilitating the shift in the burden of responsibility in effective psychotherapy, first celebrated by Roxanna Erickson-Klein's father, Milton H. Erickson, MD. The main idea is that the truly creative inner work of psychotherapy is the burden of the patient, not the therapist (*American Journal of Clinical Hypnosis*, Vol. 6, No. 3, 1964).

While popular lore tends to promote the therapist as the heroine of the psychotherapeutic encounter, there is a long tradition of innovative professionals like Colbert and Erickson-Klein introducing new attitudes and techniques for facilitating a person's own creative development in optimizing his or her own path of self-transformation and recovery. Consider how more than 100 years ago Sigmund Freud introduced free association and emphasized the patient's own dreams as harbingers of the path to self-discovery and healing. Consider how Carl Jung introduced active imagination as a key for unlocking the person's own spiritual life as an inner guide to self-fulfillment. In our time, consider how Carl Rogers introduced the simple reflection of the client's actual words and concepts as the focus for facilitating the highest levels of attention, self-understanding, and problem solving.

Colbert and Erickson-Klein now expand this innovative tradition by introducing 100 experiential activities for addiction treatment and rehabilitation. It is their emphasis on experiential novel and numinous activities that makes their approach a wonderful therapeutic application of the new neuroscience research on memory, learning, and the creation of new cognition and consciousness at the molecular-genomic level of brain plasticity and stem cell healing. Although they began this work in a local nonprofit limited to women, we can safely assume it is only the beginning of a therapeutic journey. We all look forward to the eventual extension of their creative work to all people, all cultures, and virtually all the stress-related disorders.

Ernest Lawrence Rossi, PhD

Preface

We met four years ago in an inpatient recovery setting. Kay, a Licensed Clinical Social Worker, was a member of the counseling staff and brought to the position an interest in mindful meditation. Roxanna, a Registered Nurse finishing a counseling internship, brought familiarity with clinical hypnosis and an orientation of participatory engagement. We were drawn together by our mutual interest in using experiential activities. This interest led us to develop a small notebook of ideas that we shared with other staff members about activities we had used successfully with groups. The more we worked, the more we became aware of the limitations of resource materials available for our client population. To assure we had a broad base of choices for our own use, we compiled a core collection of therapeutic activities focused on recovery skills. We sought qualitative input through scales, surveys, and discussion with other facilitators and the clients themselves. Feedback was incorporated into the activity designs. Our considerable efforts to amass a collection of useful materials eventually evolved into this book. We do not claim that all these activities are unique creations by us. Many were inspired by other sources that we modified, adapted, and updated. We have done our best to credit our inspirational bases and reference them as appropriate. What makes this collection particularly valuable is that we have tried and tested each of the activities and modified them as needed for ease of use and clarity of purpose.

The facility where we did most of our work is Nexus Recovery Center in Dallas, Texas, a well-respected, nonprofit inpatient facility that offers harbor and hope for women with active substance abuse concerns and mental health issues. Nexus is one of the few drug treatment facilities in the country that accepts pregnant women. The Nexus program uses a structured schedule, builds acceptance of personal responsibilities, and utilizes process groups, educational groups, and individual counseling. When working with groups there is the challenge, not unique to this program, to engage clients in active participation and to capture their attention in meaningful ways.

Nexus incorporates a cognitive behavioral approach and embraces twelve-step methodology, which is similar to the majority of programs offered in the United States. The center uses the broadly accepted Stages of Change model, delineated by Prochaska, Norcross, and DiClemente. Clients' readiness for change is assessed on admission, and progress is encouraged in the direction of preparation, action, and maintenance. Most of the women who spend time at Nexus have made a commitment to sobriety and enter the program while in a preparation or action phase of change. Despite the brevity of the voluntary program, the residents generally express deep appreciation for the opportunity to redirect their lives and show promising behavioral changes with insight into their addictive patterns. A structured outpatient program is offered for integrated follow-up with discharge plans that include twelve-step work, referrals for counseling, medical and mental health services, job training, and educational and housing assistance as needed.

All the activities in this book were primarily tested on clients at Nexus Recovery Center, and some of the activities were tested in other local centers. In each case, if an activity did not go smoothly, it was modified and retried. Some of the activities were additionally tested with other types of groups. It is expected that many of the activities will be useful to a broad range of individuals who can benefit from self-awareness skills, not just those in recovery from substance abuse. It is anticipated that the activities have adaptability to settings of various orientations and groups of various sizes or skill levels.

Philosophically, we present a model for self-healing designed for clients to take with them and use for ongoing support in recovery. The experiential process offers what Ernest Rossi and Kathryn Rossi in their book, *Creating New Consciousness in Everyday Life: The Psycho-Social Genomics of Self Creation,* (see Introduction) call self-generating creative moments that facilitate new consciousness.

Acknowledgments

We express grateful appreciation to:

The individuals in recovery who shared their work illustrated here.

Cindy Seamans, PhD, for her constant support and encouragement of our professional creativity.

Nexus Recovery Center for providing a safe haven for women in recovery and allowing us to be part of the miracle.

The women of Nexus who gave us open, honest feedback, and inspired our ongoing efforts.

Andrew Barroso, Olivia Klein, and Cory Shipko for their contributions.

"Life relentlessly follows you, calling on you to change your point of view, to develop a deeper understanding of yourself and life."

STEPHEN GILLIGAN

Introduction

Welcome to *Engage the Group, Engage the Brain*. We hope you find the 100 group activities to be stimulating and rewarding when you try them with your client population.

Substance abuse remains one of the most pervasive and challenging problems faced by society. Professionals who work in the recovery field have a strong desire to generate change. In many cases this passion comes from personal experience with the devastating effects substance abuse has on individuals, families, and society. The belief of those who work in this field know that it *is* possible to make a difference, which is one of the greatest assets to the process. Persistently high relapse rates are as perplexing as they are discouraging. Problems arise with lack of consistency in evaluating successful outcomes. Most studies reveal estimates of relapse rates ranging from 40–60 percent.[1,2]

The vast majority of treatment programs in the United States are based on a twelve-step methodology and utilize cognitive behavioral approaches to facilitate change. The current understanding of brain neuroplasticity has opened opportunities for a broader look at the therapeutic process and for healing by engaging the mind and body in creative ways. We are now beginning to appreciate that the incorporation of a broader base of experiential activities into treatment may be one of the keys to enhancing success in this field.

The ideology we embrace here is that recovery can be fortified through engaging clients and nurturing neuroplasticity. New associations are generated through the stimulation of becoming involved in activities that offer decision making, problem solving, and choices in a nonthreatening, supportive environment. Through healthy engagement and participation in activities that allow for expression of insight but do not require it, the individual has the opportunity to explore belonging, participation, and success in a whole different manner.

While we, the authors, support a cognitive learning foundation as centrally important to recovery, our emphasis in this book is on experiential engagement. Our activities are designed to augment and enhance existing program offerings, including those based on cognitive behavioral, Stages of Change[3], Motivational Interviewing[4], and twelve-step approaches. This is not a stand-alone approach but rather an enrichment. Not all participants are able to learn the same way or to express themselves in a traditional classroom didactic setting. Some are not able to develop insight that can be expressed verbally. Learning that is dependent upon verbal expression is limited in its reach and capacity for change.[5] We strive to go beyond the limitations of written or spoken language to reach into areas of learning that occur on an unconscious level, further than the reach of cognitive expressive learning. This book includes the application of activities that go past cognitive learning and stimulate self-reflective processes congruent with principles of neuroplasticity.

The philosophy and works of the psychiatrist Milton H. Erickson provide a framework of self-awareness and self-responsibility integral to overall health and well-being. Erickson's creative approaches to psychotherapy and speculation that his unique success may be in a tangible way related to neuroplasticity, piqued our interest in exploring neuroplasticity as a central avenue to brain health. We found the work of others who also support this concept. We share an admiration for the work of neurologist Oliver Sacks, whose many books have shown that deeper understanding of one's uniqueness is integral to health. Another book that influenced our thinking is *The Brain that Changes Itself* [6] by physician Norman Doidge, in which Doidge emphasizes the personal triumph of overcoming limitations through challenging, ingrained, habitual patterns of perception and thinking.

We draw on the work of Mindfulness Based Stress Reduction (MBSR) as it was developed by Jon Kabat-Zinn, PhD, and the Center for Mindfulness at the University of Massachusetts Medical School. Clinical research strongly supports the positive effects of MBSR, which is being integrated into other therapy protocols.[7] We are also inspired by Mindfulness-Based Relapse Prevention (MBRP), which uses empirically supported interventions developed by Alan Marlatt, Sarah Bowen, and Neeha Chawla, and others, at the University of Washington, Addictive Behaviors Research Center.

The process of brain resiliency is supported by neuroscientist Michael Merzenich, whose research at the University of California shows that the brain has the capacity to change itself in both physical and functional ways.[8] Merzenich is a leading proponent of therapeutic approaches to overcome functional limitations. These ideas are supported by a 2006 study by Dr. Sherry Willis and colleagues with the National Institute on Aging that was the first to document long-term, positive effects of cognitive training on brain function in older adults. The study showed that at nearly any point in your life, you can strengthen your brain by doing tasks that are new and complex and that stimulate a balanced variety of areas within the brain.[9]

The work of Ernest Rossi, PhD, has provided a platform from which we have designed and implemented many of our activities. Rossi posits we can enhance neural networking, stimulate dendritic growth, and promote a healthy rebalance of neurotransmitters through engaging in three areas: novelty, environmental enrichment, and physical activity. Rossi states, "Novelty, exercise, and life enrichment facilitate gene expression and brain growth."[10] He emphasizes that by pushing beyond boundaries of comfort, one can expand possibilities as well as accelerate the process of healing. Rossi has initiated supportive research, currently in progress, to document the effect of creative problem solving on genetic expression. In addition, "Gene expression and brain plasticity can consolidate the healing reconstruction of fear, stress, and traumatic memories and other symptoms in everyday life."[11]

Expression that is not limited by cognitive or verbal elements is a basic and fundamental construct of our approach. Another is being able to envision a positive future without the limitations of addiction. Elements of past, present, and future behaviors are entwined in our activities. Acceptance of what is unchangeable, learning needed skills in the present, and envisioning success in a future time are embedded lessons in most activity. In subtle ways, the activities teach learning to relax, enjoying the moment, looking at how others have fun in sober ways, recognizing that all individuals have limitations, and making associations with current capabilities that will lead to a healthy and happy future.[12]

What makes *Engage the Group, Engage the Brain* distinct is we tested each of these activities in groups with actual clients in recovery. We obtained feedback from participants and refined and adjusted activities as needed. All samples displayed in this book are the original work of clients in our groups, who graciously gave us permission to use them. The process of compiling these activities has been immeasurably rewarding for us. The clients are consistently appreciative and enthusiastic, and each session brings its own novelty and enrichment. The unexpected resourcefulness that seems to arise in nearly every session is exciting and gratifying.

It is our hope and expectation that our efforts will offer practical directions for other clinicians to feel the energy generated through this process. Science has not yet brought us to a place where we can state with certainty that these activities actually lead to neuroplasticity and help strengthen recovery; however, we offer these materials as our contribution to a promising new direction.

Introduction Notes

1. A. Thomas McLellan, David C. Lewis, Charles P. O'Brien, and Herbert D. Kleber, "Drug dependence, a chronic medical illness: Implications for treatment, insurance, and outcomes evaluation," JAMA, no. 284 (13, 2000): 1689–1695.

2. "Drug Abuse and Addiction: One of America's Most Challenging Public Health Problems," National Institute on Drug Abuse, last modified June 2005, accessed June 29, 2015. http://archives.drugabuse.gov/about/welcome/aboutdrugabuse/index.html.

3. James O. Prochaska, John Norcross, and Carlo DiClemente, *Changing for Good: A Revolutionary Six-Stage Program for Overcoming Bad Habits and Moving Your Life Positively Forward* (NewYork: Avon Books, 1994).

4. William R. Miller and Stephen Rollnick, *Motivational Interviewing: Helping People Change, Third Edition* (New York: Guiford Press, 2012).

5. Ernest L. Rossi, Roxanna Erickson-Klein, and Kathyrn L. Rossi, eds., *The Collected Works of Milton H. Erickson Volume 3: Opening the Mind* (Phoenix: Milton H. Erickson Foundation Press, 2008).

6. Norman Doidge, *The Brain that Changes Itself: Stories of Personal Triumph from the Frontiers of Brain Science* (New York: Penguin, 2007).

7. Jon Kabat-Zinn, *Full Catastrophe Living: Using the Wisdom of Your Body and Mind to Face Stress, Pain, and Illness* (New York: Delta, 2005).

8. Dean C. Buonomano and Michael M. Merzenich, "Cortical Plasticity: From Synapses to Maps," *Annual Review of Neuroscience*, no. 21 (1998), 149–86.

9. Sherry L. Willis, Sharon L. Tennstedt, Michael Marsiske, Karlene Ball, Jeffrey Elias, Kathy Mann Koepke, K. M., et al., "Long-term Effects of Cognitive Training on Everyday Functional Outcomes in Older Adults," *Journal of the American Medical Association*, no. 296 (23: 2006), 2805–2814.

10. Ernest L. Rossi and Kathyrn L. Rossi, *Creating New Consciousness in Everyday Life: The Psycho-Social Genomics of Self Creation* (Los Osos: Palisades Gateway Publishing, 2013).

11. Ibid., 964–967.

12. Philip Zimbardo, Richard Sword, and Rosemary Sword, *Time Cure: Overcoming PTSD with the New Psychology of Time Perspective Therapy* (San Francisco: Jossey-Bass, 2012).

How to Use This Book: A Facilitator's Guide

Through our experience in the field, we have learned a variety of strategies that will help you conduct dynamic groups. In this section, we share our methods for engaging participation and maximizing opportunity for therapeutic transformation.

The activities in the book may be done in any order as they might fit into your group.

Group Management: We always begin these activities with a short summary emphasizing patience, being aware of self in the present moment, and the importance of self-care. Starting with a brief review of the body's needs for a balance of nutrition, sleep, and exercise, we also emphasize a need for good spiritual and mental health. We briefly call attention to each of the six areas this book is divided into and clarify how the chosen activity relates to those areas.

We use analogies about how addiction has commonalities with other conditions. People who have brain damage from stroke, head injury, or alcohol and other drug use often have impairments in short-term memory, long-term memory, verbal or written language expression, motor skills, and emotional regulation. The concept of neuroplasticity is introduced in simple terms. Group activities are then described from the perspective of being an opportunity to enrich oneself through conditions (novelty, enrichment, and exercise) that hold promise for accelerating healing and enhancing the probability of success in recovery.

We invite participants rather than instruct, and we accept the depth and direction of engagement each participant chooses. Over and over we stress: There is no right way to do an activity; it is a process of trial and error, a discovery, a journey. We hope each person will find some aspects of the activity useful in recovery.

As clinicians and facilitators, we find it essential to stay flexible and compassionate and be willing to modify activities to suit the capabilities and moods of each particular group. One of the lessons implicit in the activities is that artistic creations rarely come out the way they are envisioned. The processes of using unfamiliar materials, making mistakes, recognizing limitations, and accepting what is imperfect are all part of what is expected. Repeatedly, we stress that it is not the product but rather the participation. The process of being expressive, creative, and challenged by a new activity is therapeutic in itself, with or without a final product. We suggest participants turn attention inward and notice what is happening in the moment (thoughts, sensations, emotions, or moods). Learning can come from handling the materials, envisioning direction, and finding a personal way to proceed. The more creative and original the direction, the more likely the participant is to make positive associations with recovery.

Participatory Reluctance: It is not unusual for individuals in inpatient treatment to ask to be excused from activities. We encourage participation, even if modified. For those less ready to adapt, individuals are encouraged to remain in groups, sit quietly, and observe what can be learned from watching others. One humorous example of how this reluctance can evolve into full participation occurred in "Exercise Circle." One participant stated she was unable to stand or exercise, so the facilitator brought her a folding chair and encouraged her to do only what was comfortable. When it was that participant's turn, she jumped up and led the group in a series of push-ups and dance moves so vigorous that few others were able to follow.

In any group, we anticipate some degree of self-consciousness or fear of participation. Certain activities involve more face-to-face contact than is comfortable for some. "Magic Hands," "Think About Me," and "Lean My Way" are among a half dozen or so activities that involve facing a partner. Some clients have stated they are uncomfortable even looking at themselves and having a partner doing the looking can be frightening or overwhelming. For these activities, we stress the voluntary nature of participation and encourage those who are not comfortable to stand back and watch the process as it evolves. Frequently, participants become more willing to explore after watching others.

The good-natured cooperative energy that evolves in groups is a powerful motivator to draw in the hesitant. One of the most delightful elements of group work is how role-modeling by some enthusiastic group members encourages participation by others, perhaps by sparking mirror neurons. For a fascinating and simple explanation of mirror neurons and brain function, we refer you to neuroscientist V.S. Ramachandran and his 2009 talk, "The Neurons that Shaped Civilization," which can be found online. Time spent observing others brings added depth and awareness. The surprising paradoxical effect of late starters becoming strong advocates is truly a beautiful process to witness.

Remarkably, cooperative sharing of skills and helping one another also tends to promote patience. One participant who had a long legal record resulting from impulsive anger management showed incredible patience in teaching others her own origami skills. She expressed insight into the change that came over her while working with the paper and began to envision how she might apply it to her own behaviors.

Holiday Blues: Holidays often bring associations with past addictive behaviors inconsistent with recovery. Engaging in appropriate, relaxing activities offers participants opportunities to begin to develop their own reservoir of happy memories associated with dates and seasons that previously created burdens. One example is St. Patrick's Day. Our activity of having each participant identify a "Hope or Dream" to display on a four-leaf clover provides a visual and emotional shift away from the commonly accepted behavior of binge drinking alcohol on that holiday. Each holiday provides opportunities to develop new associations that are pleasurable, enjoyable, and congruent with recovery.

Disparity of Skills: A broad range of abilities makes large groups challenging to work with. Some of our participants had never the learned basic skills of drawing or using scissors. Others expressed sadness over loss of skills they once had. Many comment on the limitations of their work as an indicator of how their addictions have affected them in ways in which they had not been fully aware.

In speaking with individual clients who feel their talents are limited, we counseled that those who work the hardest actually get more out of the activity than those for whom it is easy. Not everyone is artistic, and not everyone knows how to draw, cut with scissors, act, or read aloud. Not everyone is comfortable with participating in group planning. One learns from making mistakes and discovering that things often don't turn out as planned. The emphasis on self-acceptance seems to nurture a sense of hope and self-discovery despite limitations.

Materials: Many of the activities in this book require a small budget for basic arts and crafts supplies or other materials. Most of the supplies can be accumulated from households and donations. Magazines for collage, while a popular alternative to drawing images, seem to distract from intended introspection, and we strongly recommend self-generated drawing or creative designs. Some loss or theft of material supplies does occur, but this is minimal.

Samples or Mock Ups: For activities that involve some degree of performance or physical movement, we begin by asking volunteers to show the group what the activity looks like. Demonstrations are far more effective than written directions. In creating a piece of artwork, the value of having samples available is unclear. Some participants benefit from viewing samples, while others attempt to use the samples for an exact template, effectively stifling spontaneous creativity.

Time Management: Time management for some participants presents a challenge. We notice if a group member has difficulty getting started, or progresses at a pace that exceeds the time allowance, we gently call awareness to this. Keep a watchful eye on the clock to assure time is allowed both for clean-up and sharing. When using crafts materials, we eventually developed a routine of giving a ten-minute clean-up warning and allowing a limited check out of materials to conclude projects.

Clean Up: For activities that are messy or create a lot of small scraps, we used paper plates for confinement of debris. The paper plates can be reused for future projects, and interestingly, whenever they were used, some became unexpectedly incorporated into the artistic endeavors.

Adverse Reactions: In any healthcare setting, it is important to be prepared to deal with individual needs or adverse responses. Within our groups, a counselor or intern counselor is always available to deal with any needs or anxiety reactions. Nexus Recovery Center has many clients with severe trauma and PTSD, and we were always aware of the possibility of uncomfortable emotions being triggered. In fact, this happened rarely. Occasionally materials selected inadvertently caused an abreaction. One example of this was the use of India ink that reminded a client of black tar heroin. She became agitated and benefited from the presence of counseling staff. Being prepared can decrease the likelihood of such difficult situations. Subject matter that involves families could put those with significant losses or those raised in dysfunctional or foster families at risk for discomfort. Therefore, we might offer participants an alternative to describing a dream family, church family, or a family of friends. Alternative selections made are unconditionally accepted, and we see them as healthy choices in self-care.

Discussion: It is essential to allow time at the conclusion of the group for clients to present their creations and process feelings about the activity. We offered clients the opportunity to show their work to the larger group, if desired, or to keep it personal, if preferred. You will find that clients are generally enthusiastic talking about their experiences, expressing the meaning they found in the activity, and showing their artistic creations to others. Some participants want to describe ambivalence, difficulties in becoming engaged, or mistakes made. This is not discouraged, and the group forum is an effective opportunity to reframe negative thoughts in a positive way. The diversity of responses adds enormous depth. Creative ideas generated by the clients are some of the more delightful aspects of this work. All the photographs in this manual illustrate actual client work and show clinicians what results can be expected.

Thank you for selecting this book, and we hope that you find it to be useful!

Overview of the Sections

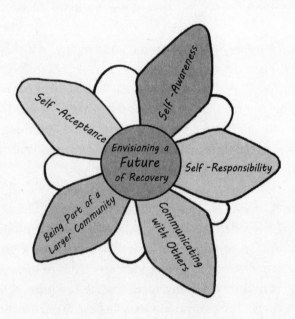

The activities in this book have been divided into six topic sections and are sequenced accordingly. The activities for each topic are listed at the beginning of that section. A complete alphabetical list of the activities is in the Appendix.

Self-Acceptance: Inventory with Unconditional Valuing of Self

Self-Awareness: Individual Strengths and Areas for Growth

Self-Responsibility: Emotional Regulation of Self Care

Communicating with Others: Expressive
Verbal and Nonverbal Connections

Being Part of a Larger Community: Participation
and Developing a Sense of Belonging

Envisioning a Future of Recovery: Anticipation
of Holidays and Success Over Time

The inpatient population in a treatment center is often fluid. Groups change from week to week, which presents challenges for group cohesion, as well as for following a sequential curriculum. In many ways, this flux mimics life and adapting to the challenge of change and uncertainty enhances the lessons implicit in this book.

These activities are not meant to be done in any particular order. This book is organized into a framework of six interconnected skill dimensions, each pertaining to essential skills of healthy living. As a facilitator, you may choose any activity that fits your timeframe or meets your needs on a particular day. At the beginning of each section, we have provided a brief overview on the particular topic, as well as additional observations from the authors.

The overall intention is to develop a constellation of skills that facilitate active participation in daily life, functionality, and appreciation for living. These activities encourage a process of learned self-correction, enabling the participant to make ongoing adjustments in life as circumstances change and grow beyond the addictive cycle. The central emphasis is on the growth process, development of internal resources, restructuring of the social context of interactions, and the building of healthy associations.

It is not uncommon to see individuals in early recovery have deficits in basic cognitive abilities. Whether necessary skills were never developed or they were impaired as a consequence of addiction, there is little doubt that skill building in this area enhances and regenerates individual growth and potential.

The activities presented here are intentionally simple and accessible. They rely on ordinary skills and knowledge and require only the most basic of learning. Yet each activity supports a process of change and is a framework upon which participants can continue to build and develop beyond the inpatient phase, beyond an interval of recovery, and in a natural trajectory that leads to sustained well-being.

Self-Acceptance: Inventory with Unconditional Valuing of Self

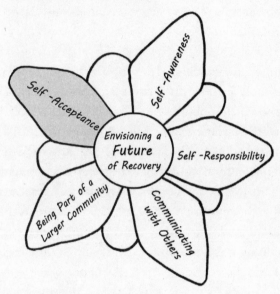

Addiction is a disorder that occurs as a result of a complex interplay of biological and genetic predispositions, coupled with environmental factors and psychosocial circumstances. Modern neuroscience shows that people with addiction and compulsive behaviors experience strong cravings that can override the rational, reflective, decision-making parts of the brain. This can explain why people with addiction often make impulsive and destructive choices in their lives that hurt themselves and the ones they love. Individuals in early recovery often have strong feelings of regret, shame, and guilt about things they have done in the past. Self-esteem and sense of self are common casualties.

Activities in this section promote an open honest self-inventory and a willingness to accept one's own history. We encourage examining the past and assessing what was painful and what was of value. Stressed in the assignments is the expectation that participants will be able to find strengths. Those very strengths are witnessed by arrival in a setting that invites recovery, despite all of the trials and hardships that may have been endured on the journey.

Roxanna: I recognize a strong need for people to have the opportunity to tell their story. As a Registered Nurse for many years, I learned patients do better if you listen to the entire story they offer rather than making assessments based on what is evidentially related to clinical symptoms. Sometimes the stories seem disjointed or irrelevant, and yet it is the internal connections that are the most relevant information of all.

While some stories seem to support tragic sequences that understandably lead to misfortune and poor life choices, other stories are completely obtuse. One adolescent with serious Obsessive Compulsive Disorder explained that a teacher had used the word *decorum* in the context of a class lecture. She attributed the teacher's use of that uncommon word to have triggered a series of life changes and lost ability to function normally. Acceptance of that strange logic was essential to her sense of being listened to, heard, respected, and treated with dignity. The validity of her commitment to the causality of her condition was not central to her health—being respected and listened to was. Once she was given the opportunity to express this association, and her story was treated with dignity, she was free to make healthier associations. Treatment and support enabled building of associations congruent with a functional future.

Kay: In the recovery community, we talk about how people with addiction are trying unsuccessfully to fill an empty hole in their soul with alcohol or other drugs. I have observed that frequently newly sober clients still feel a general sense of lack in themselves. They must now deal with a variety of uncomfortable feelings without the numbing qualities of alcohol or other drugs. David Loy, a professor of Buddhist and comparative philosophy, speaks eloquently on the sense of self and the "sense of lack" people can feel and the desire to change this by grasping at things to make them feel better, such as getting high. Those with addiction often have a sense of something not being quite right with themselves, and they look to substances to feel more secure. In recovery, one challenge is to reconstruct a healthy sense of self and to develop self-compassion and self-acceptance.

"Accept your yesterdays unconditionally. Accept your tomorrows very selectively."

Dr. Kristina Erickson

Autumn Leaves

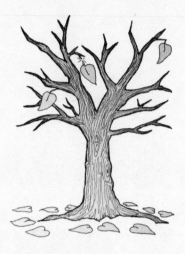

Location: Indoors

Time: 45 minutes

Materials: Construction paper (green, brown, orange, red; blue or white for background)

Removable sticky tape, glue dots, glue, or glue sticks

Markers

Scissors

Optional: leaf shapes for templates

Objectives

- To stimulate thinking about behaviors, habits, or experiences that clients are ready to let go.

- To provide a visual representation of the process and a way to self-check desired changes.

Directions

1. Review directions and anticipated outcome with the group.

2. Ask each participant to choose a background sheet of construction paper.

3. Instruct participants to design their own tree trunk out of brown construction paper.

4. Have them cut out leaf shapes and glue them onto the branches of the tree.

5. Direct participants to place a few leaves at the base of the tree.

6. Tell participants to set aside four or five leaves on which to identify some personal feeling or behavior that one wishes to "leave behind."

7. On the selected leaves, have participants write specific behaviors they wish to overcome. For example, snacking excessively, chewing fingernails, being impatient, procrastinating, or being late for appointments.

8. Using removable tape, have participants place the selected leaves on the tree or falling toward the ground. They can be positioned with the behavior showing or turned privately inward.

9. Encourage participants to keep the tree, and as they make progress, move the leaves down toward the ground.

10. If desired, paricipants can write behaviors of the past that they have already left behind on the fallen leaves.

Observations

This activity was done with a group of twelve. Several participants needed help and individualized attention to get started and to conceptualize desired life change. All embraced the concept of identifying behaviors they wished to leave behind, and about half put their trees in strategic locations so they could do daily checkups. One woman made a Christmas tree and decorated it with pinecones that fell off—Christmas represented her target date for achieving the desired changes.

Inspired by: A Yaqui Indian ceremony in which the entire village lets go of personal issues and the entire village is cleansed in a group ceremony.

Childhood Comforts

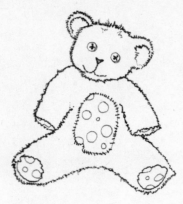

Location: Indoors

Time: 35 minutes

Materials: Jumbo pencils and crayons, the style used in early elementary school

Construction paper

Objectives

- To encourage positive recollection of and appreciation of internal resources.
- To access the creative resourcefulness of childhood.

Directions

1. Invite participants to recall the variety of ways in which each found safety as a child, with emphasis on the child's adaptive wit. Emphasize the unexpected multitude of creative ways children have in recognizing and attending to the need for comfort.

2. Read aloud the following explanation:
This activity is designed to bring out the remembrances of when you were young and looked forward to the time when you could have a 32- or 64-pack of crayons. But back then, you learned to adapt and to work with the colors at hand.
The purpose of using elementary school materials is to bring back a time when participants faced challenges different from the ones they experience as adults. Note that the jumbo crayons come in only eight colors.

3. Encourage discussion within the group of possible responses: a place, gesture, toy, pet, relationship, or activity. There is no correct discovery.

4. Emphasize that this is neither an art project nor an evaluation of artistic ability. It will not be graded or displayed. It is a process of self-discovery.

5. Remind participants they can use as many sheets of paper as needed.

6. Invite participants to make an artistic rendering or a symbol of something that brought comfort to them as a child. Read aloud the following explanation: *No matter what our background as children, each of us went through normal, healthy developmental stages in which we discovered our own ways of finding resources to help us feel safe or comforted. The purpose*

*of this activity is to remember some strengths and resources
we discovered in childhood and to capture and enjoy those
feelings. In this safe environment, where we are here and now,
remember a time when you were very young. You are invited
to close your eyes and think back to ways that you found safety
and comfort as a child. Maybe it was a friend, pet, toy, doll, a
stuffed animal, a blanket, or some other object. Or maybe it
was a hiding place or secret playhouse where you learned to feel
safe and comfortable in your own way, all on your own. Use the
materials here to draw those images, which is a way to help you
to remember some of the strengths that have kept you safe.*

7. Invite volunteers to show their work and talk about the meaning.

Observations

By encouraging recollection and appreciation of resources within, the client is better equipped to problem solve in the present and future. This strength-based activity encourages connection to forgotten or unappreciated internal resources. A study by Sarah Davies and Gail Kinman, presented in 2010 at the British Psychological Society's Annual Conference, indicated that recovering alcoholics who focus on positive experiences in their past may be more successful in managing their addiction.

This activity was performed in a cafeteria setting on two separate occasions. Several group members had come from traumatic life circumstances and had never had a healthy or safe home life. Permission was given to draw what they felt like. Initially, two group members were withdrawn, but as the drawing began, everyone became more expressive. Some reassurance was needed regarding poor drawing ability. Both occasions resulted in full participation—everyone became actively engaged and wanted to tell the group about their drawings.

The range of responses included special blankets and a dog who "listened"; several participants cited a grandmother, an aunt, a neighbor, and stuffed toys or dolls. One of the women who had lived in a series of foster homes found comfort in church and drew the gesture of her foster mother looking over her shoulder to see she was sitting in the pew behind. Without exception, the activity was received in a positive manner. The discussion among group members was powerful and memorable. Being able to connect with any sense of safety was considered a benefit.

Art therapy attributes meaning to layers and individual interpretation of designs. While this activity was not done as art therapy, those elements were recognized and therapeutically discussed with participants.

Inspired by: This activity was designed after watching a group of elementary school children drawing their own safe places. The enthusiasm of the youngsters and their adaptability to circumstance was remarkable.

"The process of growth that accompanies a relaxing exercise fills in some pieces that were missed in childhood."

ROXANNA ERICKSON-KLEIN

Family Tree

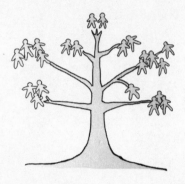

Location: Indoors

Time: 60 minutes

Materials: Pens or pencils

Blank paper

Family tree handouts

Samples based on the templates

Objectives

- To offer a multigenerational perspective on various qualities or characteristics found in families, including mental illness or substance use.

- To facilitate identification of risk factors.

- To encourage change.

Directions

1. Before the session begins, review the suggested templates and create samples to show. Alternatives are shown for a traditional family, a modified family, and a foster family.

2. Introduce participants to the concept of charting family trees.

3. Explain a simple family tree using a three- or four-generation format.

4. Engage participants in discussion of visible physical traits that can be identified through generations, such as eye color.

5. Identify patterns of behavior that are seen through generations, such as occupations, hobbies, or religious affiliation.

6. Discuss potential for behavioral patterns, including substance abuse, mental illness, or domestic violence to occur in multiple generations.

7. Facilitate group discussion identifying the value of raising awareness of patterns.

8. Direct participants to create their own multigenerational family tree and illustrate how various traits or qualities may be expressed over the generations.

9. Encourage participants to share feelings, discoveries, or self-understandings gained from the activity.

Observations

This activity was performed twice with groups of eight and ten members. Of those present, few had ever explored their own backgrounds in this manner. Qualities in addition to substance use that were discussed included musical ability, sickle cell disease, hypertension, family size, living to old age, and being accident prone. Participants responded with seriousness, and most stated that they expect to continue exploration into this aspect of their lives. One woman knew little of her biological family, had lived in foster homes, and charted a family of friends. Several of the participants required assistance in getting started with the chart development. Be prepared to provide comfort or grounding to those who start grieving loss of family or dysfunctional familial connections. It can be affirming to recognize that everyone does not come from a traditional family system.

Inspired by: The work of Monica McGoldrick, LCSW, PhD (h.c.), Director of the Multicultural Family Institute in Highland Park, New Jersey. This activity is superficial compared to her more serious works.

Foster Family Tree

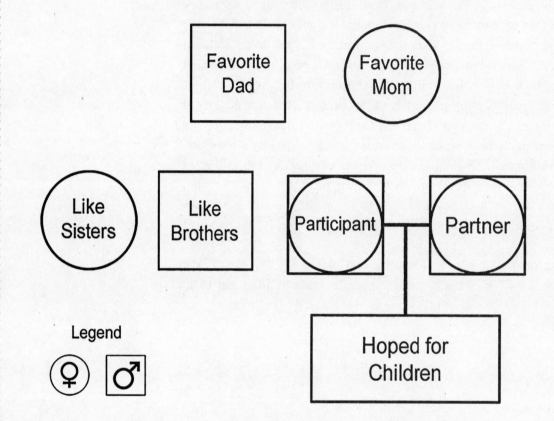

Traditional Family Tree

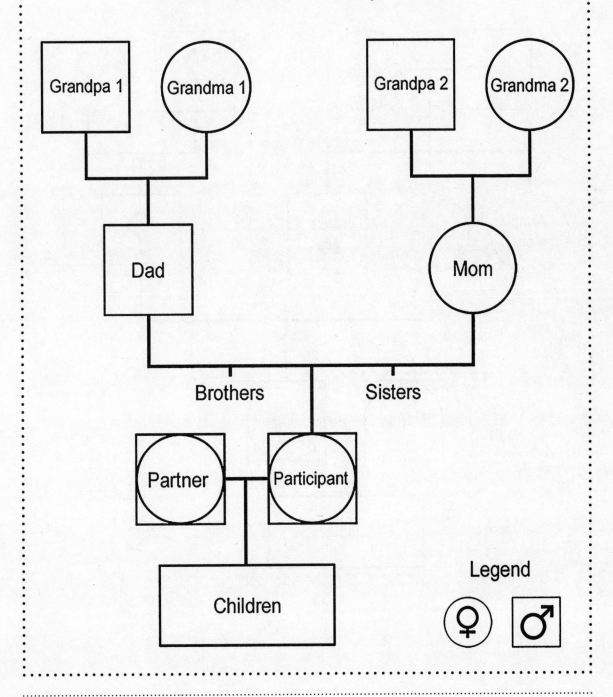

Modified Family Tree

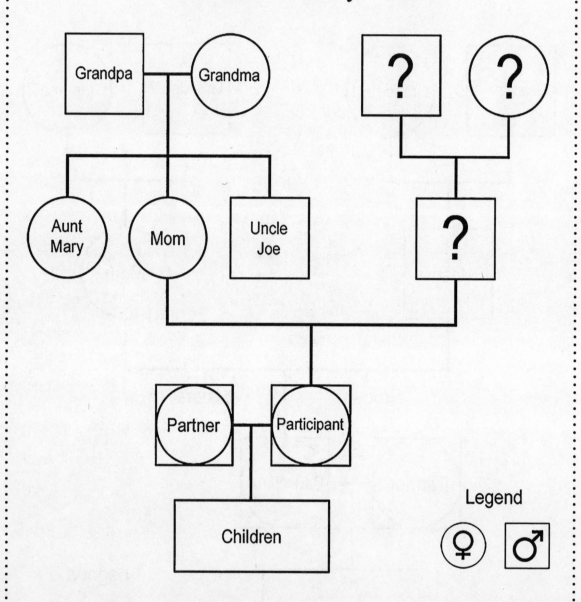

Legend

"Bear in mind that we have a wealth of ways of escaping that are normal."

Milton H. Erickson

Gratitude Books

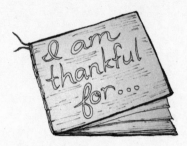

Location: Indoors

Time: 60–90 minutes

Materials: Colored paper

Writing paper

Decorative or scrapbook paper

Card stock

Markers, pencils, or pens

Scissors

Glue

Stapler

Ribbons or strings

Optional: holiday template shapes

Objectives

- To have a positive thinking activity that could be used on holidays or times when clients tend to feel restless and discontent.

- To shift the focus from resentment in the twelve-step tradition to that of gratitude, counteracting self-pity and negative thinking.

Directions

1. Prepare a sample book in advance to show group.

2. Show group the sample book and explain the activity.

3. Discuss possible moments of gratitude in participants' lives to include in their book.

4. Invite participants to choose materials from the available supplies. Any size or shape book of approximately six pages can be constructed from card stock and writing paper. It can be decorated with craft materials, recovery slogans, drawings, or collage materials. To tie it in to a particular holiday, you can use templates of shapes, such as hearts for Valentine's Day, turkeys for Thanksgiving, and pumpkins for Halloween.

5. Once clients have completed their books, suggest they write about their moments of gratitude on the pages. If they wish, they can pass their books around for other people to write something positive or encouraging about them.

6. Encourage participants to share their finished products.

Observations

Everyone was enthusiastic about this simple activity. Often the activity took place on holiday weekends when regular programming was flexible. Participants were often reflective about missing their families and loved ones, and sometimes the longing for family prompted the impulse to consider leaving treatment early. This activity provided a useful and productive redirection that was engaging and affirming and enhanced twelve-step work.

Inspired by: Staff at the center where we worked always noted increases in depression, anxiety, and restlessness around holidays, and this activity was developed to address the issue.

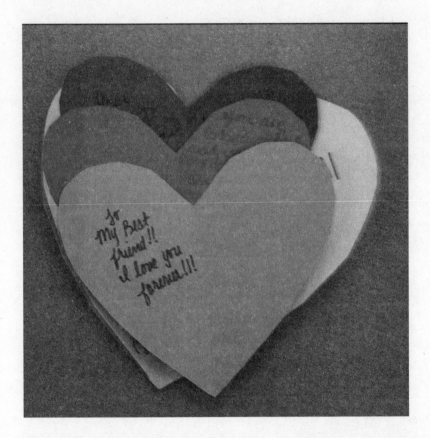

This heart-shaped gratitude book that was passed around for encouraging comments from peers. One inscription reads, "For My Best friend!! I love you forever!!!" Another says, "You are so beautiful and so is your spirit!"

Human Bingo

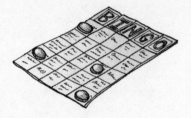

Location: Indoors or Outdoors

Time: 15–20 minutes depending on number of participants

Materials: Human Bingo Handout (one per person)

Pen or pencil (one per person)

Small prizes for each win (candies, pens, stickers, or writing paper)

Objectives

- To promote healthy social skills and listening skills.
- To display the variety of talents and strengths of individuals.

Directions

1. Make copies of the Bingo cards. You may modify questions as needed.

2. Pass out the writing materials and the Bingo cards. A Bingo may depend on the size of the particular group. With a large number of people, you may ask that all squares be signed. Or, you may decide that any number of rows (diagonal, horizontal, vertical) may provide a win. Read the instructions aloud:

   Find someone who has ever done or can do the thing described in each square.

   Have this person sign the square.

   Bingo wins!

   Now go talk to each other!

Observations

This activity was done outside on a nice day and was an enjoyable warm-up. It was repeated at another type of rehabilitation center with equally positive results.

Inspired by: Icebreaker activities done in social work graduate school at the University of Texas at Arlington and the popularity of Bingo games in the treatment center.

Human Bingo HANDOUT

Find someone who has done these things and have him or her sign the square.

Free Space	Watched Sesame Street	Has Moved More than 5 Times	Can Do the Splits	Makes Pizza from Scratch	Has Been Scuba Diving	Broken an Arm or Leg	Been to a Pro Basketball Game
Has a Motorcycle	Favorite Color Is Green	Grew Up in a Very Small Town	Likes Sushi	Born Same Month as You	Has at least 5 Traffic Tickets	Can Do a Cartwheel	Has a Facebook Page
Knows How to Do the Harlem Shake	Has Eaten an Insect or Worm	Is Left Handed	Can Juggle	Has Performed on Stage	Overdrew a Checking Account	Is a Vegetarian	Born Outside the USA
Is a Morning Person	Can Speak Another Language	Plays Guitar	Likes Salty over Sweet	Sings in the Shower	Has Read More than 30 Books	Been to a Pro Baseball Game	Has Same Number of Siblings as You
Has Been Rock Climbing	Changed a Diaper	Has Parachuted or Bungee'd	Is an Only Child	Can Tell a Funny Joke to You	Been to California	Has 4 or More Pets	Has Run a 10K or Marathon
Has Milked a Cow	Has Been to a Pro Football Game	Has Used an Outhouse	Has Marched in a Parade	Can Touch Tongue to Nose	TP'd a House	Knows a Celebrity	Is a Parent or Legal Guardian
Is a Cat Person	Has a Scar Over 3 Inches Long	Has a Secret Tattoo	Has a Hole in Sock Now	Played Competitive Soccer	Has Been Ice Skating	Was a Girl or Boy Scout	Was Suspended from School
Likes to Go Camping	Is a Dog Person	Likes to Swim	Has Slept in Church	Has Been White Water Rafting	Played the Lottery	Loves Chocolate	Likes to Ride Horses

I Am: A Poem About Myself

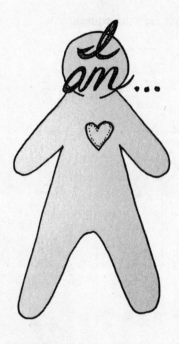

Objectives

- To increase a sense of self-awareness in the present moment.

Directions

1. In a quiet setting, encourage participants to use the opportunity to self-reflect and compose comments about themselves that are both truthful and positive. For those who are having a good day, it is reflected in the ideas. For those who struggle, it takes some extra effort but can bring out a feeling of hope and purpose.

2. Pass out a sheet of paper and the I Am Handout as a poem template for each line, which can be adapted by participants.

3. Encourage volunteers to share their poems.

Observations

This activity was done twice in groups of twelve to sixteen. Most read their poems to the group, who had touching and heartfelt responses. All participants kept their poems and expressed pride in their work.

Inspired by: A website for educators produced by the Educational Technology Training Center. They have numerous templates to help write "instant poetry" created by Alysa Cummings, Certified Poetry Therapist.

Location: Indoors or Outdoors

Time: 60 minutes

Materials: Writing paper

I Am Handout (one per person)

Optional: Decorative materials

I am determined + hopeful
I wonder if I'll fully recover
I hear my H.Power
I see my future ahead of me.

I pretend ~~feel~~ that I see his face
I feel the emptiness inside
I touch my soul again
I worry that i'll fall
I cry ~~about~~ at all I gave up good + bad
I am determined + hopeful

I understand that I must Faith
I say every relapse gets worse
I dream to find healthy love
I try to do what's right
I hope for no more pain
I am determined + hopeful

Sample poem that demonstrates personal creativity with the format.

I Am HANDOUT

Use these sentence stems to write a poem about yourself.

I am _____ (two or three words to describe you)

I awoke this morning _____ (two words of description)

I found myself _____ (where or feeling how)

I saw something _____ (normal or unusual)

I thought about _____ (something good)

That reminds me of _____ (something that is good)

I am _____ (repeat the first line of your poem)

I believe in _____ (a feeling word or phrase)

I want to believe in _____ (something you question but hope for)

I know that _____

I hope that _____

I am sure about _____

I am _____ (repeat the first line of your poem)

I already _____ (something you are doing)

I will learn to _____ (something you are working toward)

I am moving _____

As I _____

I will be _____

I am _____ (repeat the first line of your poem)

Sample poem that follows the provided format.

I am a Mother myself.
I woke up this morning missing my Mom.
I found myself remembering things she did for me.
I saw that I had forgotten that she died a long time ago.
I thought about keeping her alive within me.
That reminds me of how important it is to be the Mom I want to be.
I am a Mother myself.
I believe my children are a gift from God.
I want to believe I am worthy.
I know that I love my children.
I hope that they know that I do.
I'm sure about the love that I feel.
I am a Mother myself.
I already send my love.
I will learn to let them have space to grow apart.
I am moving through time.
As I grow in God.
I will be loved.
I am a Mother myself.

Images of Belonging

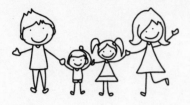

Location: Indoors or Outdoors

Time: 60 minutes

Materials: A designated "stage" area observable by the audience

Optional: list of potential poses for the actors

Objectives

- To bring internally held images into the open.

- To represent a social constellation from the participants' past, present, or future.

- To create a "snapshot" of a family or identity group using the media of "actors."

- To better understand internally held images and work beyond them.

Directions

1. Have a cofacilitator monitor activity and provide grounding in case anyone begins to find the activity upsetting or is triggered by a past trauma.

2. Introduce the purpose of the activity.

3. Review the terms used in the activity.

   - Stage: the end of the room visible to the audience

   - Audience: all group members with the exception of the artist

   - Artist: the individual in charge of creating the sculpture—a rotating role

   - Actors: two to five audience members selected by the artist to pose in the sculpture

   - Sculpture: the art generated by the artist as he or she poses the various actors

4. As a demonstration, compose your family of origin sculpture using participants as actors. For example, the actor representing father is posed as Statue of Liberty, and the actor representing mother is posed in adoration. Actors representing multiple siblings are posed in closeness to mother. The artist is represented by actor holding on to father's shirttails.

5. Describes the actors and what they represent.

6. Select a volunteer artist to demonstrate his or her sculpture.

   - Artist chooses first actor and positions, beginning the sculpture.

   - Artist selects second actor and positions.

   - Artist chooses third actor and positions.

   - Artist continues positioning actors until the sculpture is complete. Do not use more than half the number of people in the room. Most sculptures involve no more than three to four actors. One actor, for example, may represent a group or class of people, parents, or siblings.

   - Once the sculpture is complete, artist turns to the audience and describes the work.

   - On completion, the actors return to their seats ready for the next artist demonstration.

7. Have all group participants take a turn being the artist, demonstrating their sculpture.

8. A second round of demonstrations may be desired in which an identity group is used instead of the family origin, such as a workplace, a group of friends, or a support group. The artist repeats steps as demonstrated previously, using group members to construct the new sculpture.

9. Once each participant has demonstrated their sculpture, initiate a discussion about any of the works presented.

10. Conclude with a debriefing process to put matters into current perspective.

Observations

This activity was performed twice with groups of eight and ten. In each group, a member was present who had been raised in foster homes, but each adapted quickly to the suggestion of choosing one family to represent. The facilitator's demonstration of her own family image proved to be a powerful stimulus to engagement, and all group members participated enthusiastically. The discussion that followed each of the demonstrations revealed a good deal of feelings held within and opened channels for working through unacknowledged emotions. During the discussion phase, it was necessary to emphasize identifying actors by their actual names: "She's not really your mother, she's Judy." The potential list of actor poses were developed after the first session to facilitate imagery and used by only a few of the participants. There was a tendency to use a tall, stately woman as the father image and a tiny young woman as the child in all the sculptures. This repeated choice of actors was acknowledged in the concluding discussion. In both sessions, the activity was universally well-received and described as powerful and helpful by the clients.

Potential actor poses suggested by group members:

Grizzly Bear	Statue of Liberty	Protective Shield
Rag Doll	The Children	Baby Bird
Mad Dog	Door Mat	Running Away
In Hiding	Helping Hand	In Adoration
In the Middle	Looking Away	Nowhere Near

Inspired by: The pioneering influence of psychodrama by Jacob Moreno has been a source of significance in this form of expression. It was, however, Virginia Satir's work in family sculpting and teaching by counselor Lilian Borges, who integrates body sculpting in her therapeutic approaches that inspired development of this activity.

"The most valuable teaching comes from the members of the group, not the facilitator."

KAY COLBERT

Letter to Me

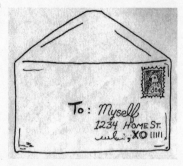

Location: Indoors

Time: 30–45 minutes

Materials: Pens

Paper or assortment of stationery (some with lines)

Envelopes

Stamps

Optional: Letter to Me Handout (one per person)

Objectives

- To project oneself in a positive future.

- To reinforce appropriate self-supportive behavior.

Directions

1. Discuss writing a letter to oneself. This letter will have advice the client would like to give him- or herself in the future. Review a list of potential topics for the letters. These might include positive reinforcing feelings, observations, reassurance, recollections, reminders, things learned in treatment, or affirmations.

2. Have participants compose a personal letter, not to be shared with the group, to give themselves supportive feedback and encouragement.

3. Ask participants to address the letter to themselves, sign it, and date it with today's date.

4. Gather letters and mail them at a future date. This can be a few days after the individual leaves residential treatment or in a few weeks.

Observations

This activity was conducted several times, with and without the handout and with and without fancy stationery. It was so well received that stationery, cards, and stamps are kept on hand as a special reward to those who have exceeded performance. A variation for this activity is to construct a "Time Capsule of Letters" that are held for thirty days prior to mailing.

Inspired by: The satisfaction of getting personal mail.

Letter to Me HANDOUT

Questions to Consider When Writing Letter to Self

What would you like to say to your future self about your recovery?

What are four reasons you should avoid alcohol or other drugs?

What advice can you give yourself about what to do if you feel like using?

What do you want your future self to be like a year from now?

What dreams and goals do you have for yourself?

What would you like to accomplish in life? Think about your personal life, career, finances, love, health, and personal growth.

What positive change would you like to see in yourself?

What will help you to cope with difficulties?

What are three things you can say to encourage yourself if you get down?

Mantra

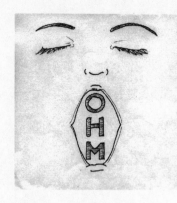

Location: Indoors

Time: 30 minutes

Materials: 3" × 5" index cards

Drawing paper

Pens, pencils, or markers

Optional: decorating materials

Mantra Handout (one per person)

Objectives

- To find a simple, yet personally meaningful, word that one can intentionally return to as a reminder to stay in recovery.

- To develop an additional coping skill to manage anxiety.

Directions

1. Discuss briefly that there are many ways we can focus and manage stress, anxiety, or cravings.

2. Invite participants to turn their attention inward to explore various ways in which a single word or mantra can resonate in a lasting way. Explain that mantras are words or phrases that are chanted aloud or to oneself to help with grounding, calming, or meditation. Offer some examples, such as *ohm* or *Follow your path* to the group so they can better understand what is expected.

3. Ask participants to think of a word that can quickly and easily remind them of their own inner strength to maintain recovery.

HOPE mantra

4. Instruct participants to write their chosen mantra on an index card and then illustrate a larger image to share with the group.

5. Once everyone is finished, invite volunteers to share their work with the group.

Observations

Initially, individuals in the group had some difficulties understanding the concept but with some explanation, the concept became simple. Each participant was invited to explain which word she chose, many of which were individual in nature. One participant described her mantra as "pull out," the place on the road to stop a runaway truck, and explained how focusing on that phrase would intercept her potential relapse. Another participant created the word *order* out of letters that spelled *chaos*. Overall, the activity was surprising, entertaining, and pleasant. Six months later, in a chance encounter, one client stated this had helped her avoid relapse. The Mantra Handout was created by clients in one of the groups.

Inspired by: Eastern meditation practices and grounding activities.

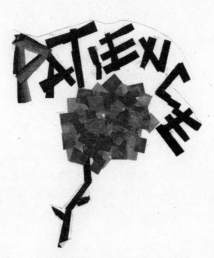

PATIENCE mantra

Mantra HANDOUT

Use one of these personal mantra suggestions or create your own.

ability	castle	driver	guardian
achievement	center	expect	guidance
ambition	change	faith	happiness
beauty	choice	freedom	help
becoming	clean	God	hope
beginning	conviction	good	human
Bible	definitely	grace	judgment
birth	dream	gift	commitment
Lord	receive	start	understanding
peace	relief	steward	win
phoenix	right	today	wish
present	rise	transformation	won
prayer	smart	truth	yes
protection	spirit	trust	

"The exercises provide a healthy and playful opportunity for self-discovery."

ROXANNA ERICKSON-KLEIN

Picture of My Addiction

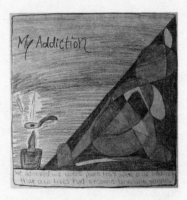

Location: Indoors (need tables for participants to work on)

Time: 90 minutes

Materials: Large drawing paper

Pens, markers, or colored pencils

Colored construction paper and/or scrapbook paper

Magazines

Craft supplies

My Addiction Handout (one per person)

Objectives

- To encourage people to describe their addiction to alcohol or other drugs in more concrete, rather than general, terms.

- To help individuals explore aspects of their addiction they do not want to give up, as well as those they do.

Directions

1. Review directions on Picture of My Addiction Handout.

2. Emphasize that each person can tell his or her story and share it in a safe, nonjudgmental environment.

Observations

This is a simple, yet effective, method to help participants begin to share personal stories. The hands-on approach can help participants, who are unable to find the words, to describe what they want to communicate. Others in the group find comfort in shared experiences and can learn from peers.

Inspired by: A similar activity seen during a professional training at the Betty Ford Center in Rancho Mirage, California.

Picture of My Addiction HANDOUT

Draw or use images to create a picture of your addiction.

Use your imagination to describe and show a picture of how you use, what substances you use, any feelings or events that usually cause you to use, and any feelings you have when you use alcohol or other drugs. You will present your picture to the group.

Here is one example just to give you an idea. Use markers, pens, and photos or words from magazines to create your picture. Make sure it fits on one sheet of paper. Be creative!

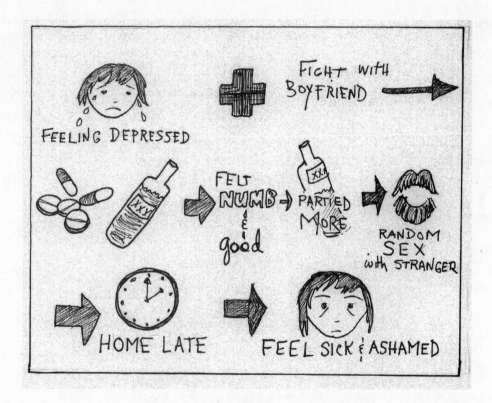

Pop-Out Messages

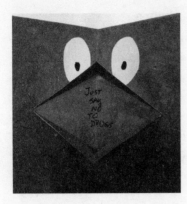

Location: Indoors

Time: 90 minutes

Materials: Construction paper

Glue

Colored markers

Scissors

Sample pop-out message

Optional: list of positive affirmations (see Appendix)

Objectives

- To provide positive affirmations in a creative manner that will help clients, or their loved ones, abstain from using alcohol and other drugs.

Directions

1. Before the session, construct a sample to show the group. As an option, create a list of positive affirmations to put in the books.

2. Begin with scratch paper to learn how to construct the pop out feature.

3. Take two sheets of paper that are different colors, but the same size.

4. Fold both papers in half to form a card.

5. Cut a slit perpendicular to the seam of the inner sheet, about two-thirds of the way across the card.

6. Lay the inner sheet with the slit in it on a flat surface, and turn back the folded edges of the slit forming a triangle on the seam side of the closed card. Fold frontward and backward to soften the fold.

7. Fold flat so the inside sheet again looks like a rectangle with a slit on the fold side. The fold marks will create two triangles from the end of the slit to the fold.

8. Mark the width and height of the mouth on the outer sheet. Write a positive affirmation within that space on the outer sheet.

9. Open the inner sheet. Gently push the two triangles in the opposite direction and fold them so the triangles appear on the inside of the folded rectangle. This will construct a pop-out mouth within the inner sheet of the card.

10. Glue outside sheet and inside sheet together. Do not place any glue underneath the pop-out mouth.

11. Decorate as desired.

Observations

A number of the participants made cards for their children, most with "Say No to Drugs" and a few with "I Love You" as the message. This was done in a group of thirty-two over a holiday weekend, and almost all expressed gratitude for having the opportunity to relax and enjoy the activity. The only difficult step is the reverse triangle fold, which several of the participants were able to do without difficulty and teach to others.

Inspired by: An activity done in an elementary school class.

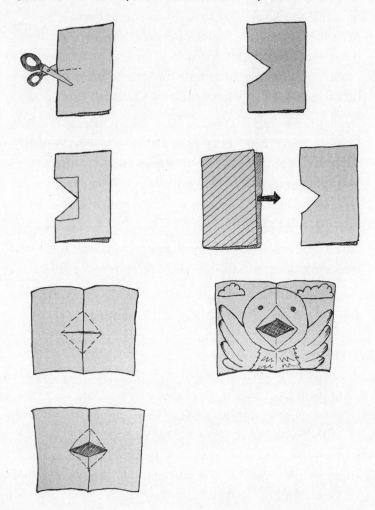

Power Animals

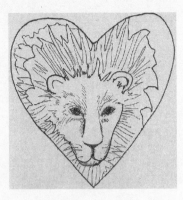

Location: Indoors or Outdoors

Time: 45 minutes

Materials: Animal pictures from magazines, a sets of stickers or clip art

Construction paper

Glue

Colored markers

Optional: Activity can be completed without pictures or art supplies, using verbal skills and imagination.

Objectives

- To cultivate inner power.

- To identify personal features that represent strength and positive attributes. To explore the diversity of individual spirit.

Directions

1. Introduce the concept that each person holds within resources and connections with other people and other animals. Some cultures recognize a special connection between animal and human, and in some settings that relationship is considered to be lifelong. You may wish to discuss traditional Native American beliefs about animal totems as a creative starting point. Emphasize that this activity offers an opportunity to reach beyond a pleasant memory or favorite pet into deeper held perspectives on what represents strength.

2. Display the animal images and art supplies. Invite participants to select from the photographs available, or to describe their animals. The animal can be real or imaginary, one that the participants have had contact with or only dreamed about. Emphasize there are no correct answers, and no animal is more positive than another.

3. Direct participants to add words around their selected animal image that describe how the animal represents strength.

4. Encourage participation in a discussion about the participants' animals and their rationale behind the selections.

Observations

A group of twelve women selected from photographs from magazines. Two of the women selected dogs, animals that had been significant in their childhood, one of whom wrote a three-page, heartfelt narrative telling of the bond she shared with her dog. One woman chose a scorpion and justified it with appropriate observations and insight regarding the strengths of this creature. All participants readily shared their selections and spoke with reverence while describing the felt connection. Others in the group identified a horse, a giraffe, a lion, an arctic tern, and a hummingbird. Each description showed contemplative resourcefulness and was received with respect by other group members. In the professional group where one author was first introduced to this activity, one man selected the cockroach as his power animal and explained in a convincing way that the insects had inhabited the earth longer than any other species and had shown unparalleled resiliency in survival. Unusual individual connections, such as the cockroach or the scorpion, must be received with as much respect as the obvious or more appealing symbols.

Inspired by: Larry Dossey, MD, discussed this at a professional meeting decades ago; we subsequently encountered variations in a number of settings and created our own adaptation.

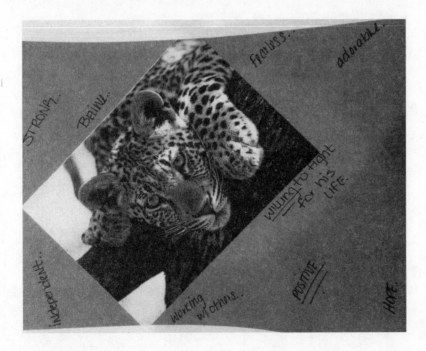

The leopard is seen as brave, strong, fearless, independent, and willing to fight for his life.

Sensory Exercise

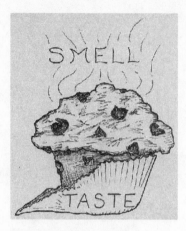

Location: Indoors (a space where participants can sit in circle)

Time: 30 minutes

Materials: Sensory Exercise Handout (for facilitator)

Objectives

- To facilitate one's agility in accessing sights, sounds, images, pictures, and associations with internal feelings of peace and beauty.

- To strengthen the sensory register, which serves as a bridge from short-term to long-term memory.

Directions

1. Describe the purpose of the activity and the way it will proceed.

2. Encourage participants to use their senses of sight, smell, taste, touch, and hearing to access mental images. The images can be from the present, remembered from the past, or live in the imagination.

3. As each participant describes the imagery, instruct others in the group to use their imagination to experience those images in their own mind.

4. Select two volunteers for a short demonstration to the group.

   - Facilitator: *In the first round, we will use our sense of sight to notice things in the surroundings that are red, or things that you remember seeing that are red.*

   - Volunteer #1: *I see a red shirt.*

   - Volunteer #2: *I remember red hot candy.*

   - Facilitator: *That's good; now use the sense of smell and the color orange.*

   - Volunteer #1: *I remember the smell of orange blossoms.*

   - Volunteer #2: *I can remember the smell of a tangerine that has just been peeled.*

5. Chooses a sensory channel and a color for each round.

6. Go around the circle, not moving too quickly, but encouraging participants to take the time to savor the images. The slower, more deliberate, and more expressive the participants are willing to be, the more that will be gained through the activity.

7. Have participants share at least ten expressions of one sensory channel-color combination prior to changing the channel or color.

Observations

The sensory register is associated with our senses—seeing (visual), hearing (auditory), moving (kinesthetic), feeling (tactile), and smelling (olfactory). The sensory register is involved in memories that last briefly, perhaps a few seconds or a few minutes, but are then forgotten. This activity was performed twice, once with a group of thirty-five and once with a group of twenty-two. With the larger group, it was markedly more difficult to engage the group, and several participants were unable to maintain the focus on sense and/or color. In the group of twenty-two, there was a greater awareness of the categorical designations and effort to comply with rotations. In the days following the activity, several women from the smaller group reported they had adapted the process into a bedtime relaxation exercise.

Inspired by: Childhood games with siblings.

Sensory Exercise HANDOUT

1. Think about:

Your current surroundings

Your memories

Your imagination

What is in your future?

2. Using one sensory modality:

Sight

Hearing

Smell

Touch

Taste

Temperature

3. Using one color:

Red

Orange

Yellow

Green

Blue

Indigo

Violet

Brown

Black

Gray

White

Clear

"Experience is the only teacher."

MILTON H. ERICKSON

Story of Your Name

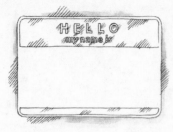

Location: Indoors

Time: 45 minutes

Materials: Blank name tags

Plastic sleeves for tags

Markers

Construction paper or craft paper

Stationery

Optional: envelopes, stamps

Objectives

- To strengthen one's sense of self-identity in a positive way.

Directions

1. Have participants decorate a wearable name tag.

2. Direct participants to write a letter of appreciation to someone who was involved in naming them. This could be their mother, whomever they were named after, or perhaps someone who has made them feel good about their name in the past.

3. Ask participants to address the group with a short presentation about his or her name. In the presentation, participants should describe if they were named after someone or have a nickname and reflect on the suitability of the given name.

Observations

This activity was done in a group of thirty-seven. Most replaced the plain standard issue name tags with brightly decorated, cheerful tags. Writing letters was an optional activity but turned out to be the most appreciated segment of the session. These letters may be mailed or not, as appropriate for each group member. In the presentation segment, many read the letters of appreciation they had written. Contents of the letters ranged from, "I never told you before about how proud I am to be named after you" to "Thank you for choosing my name even though I go by my nickname." Several people noted they had never let their aunts, who they were named after, know the kinship they felt. One woman was named after a stranger whom her mother met in the hospital and spoke good-naturedly about how unprepared for motherhood her mother must have felt at the time. Many told family tales about combining names to come up with just the right sound. Several knew nothing about their name and were then encouraged to reflect on their own feelings. None of the women had negative comments about their names.

Inspired by: The women in treatment talking about the history of their own names.

"Start with who you are today
and go from there."

Roxanna Erickson-Klein

Timelines

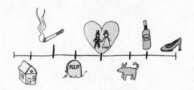

Location: Indoors (the area needs to have tables)

Time: 90 minutes

Materials: Rolls of newsprint paper (cut into approximately 60 inches per person)

Pens, markers, or colored pencils

Collage paper

Decorative materials

Magazines

Rulers

Scissors

Timelines Handout

Objectives

- To encourage participants to reflect on significant moments in their lives and begin to make connections or observe patterns.

- To identify cause and effect.

- To put life events (including substance abuse and mental health issues) into context and perspective.

Directions

1. Distribute Timelines Handout. Instruct participants to include positive or negative events. They should try to identify at least five or six life events that stand out to them. If participants have blank spots in their memory, reassure them this is fine and have them note what comes to mind.

2. Have volunteers pass out newsprint. Place art supplies on the tables.

3. Direct participants to draw a large timeline on their newsprint and transfer the events on their handout to the newsprint. Encourage them to decorate the events—using pictures instead of words is acceptable. Assure everyone there is no right or wrong way to do the activity.

4. Give positive feedback as participants work. From time to time, alert them to how much time they have left.

5. When everyone is done, have participants share their timeline with the group, explaining their life story as much as they are comfortable. Promote a discussion about what was thought of while each person was creating the timeline and if connections were made.

Observations

This activity was done over a dozen times. While a few participants may finish quickly, most will need sixty to ninety minutes. Some may keep the timelines and add to them in their free time. Each time, there were several people who spontaneously discovered repeating patterns of behavior. It was common for those who had significant traumas in their lives to have periods of memory loss. The facilitator should be prepared to normalize this experience and encourage them to leave a small blank space and move on. Participants who suffer from more severe mental illness or cognitive impairments may not be able to follow the chronological pattern, but they can be encouraged to draw or collage what they remember. Most enjoyed sharing their finished timelines and often displayed them in their rooms. For the facilitator, it was helpful to see an illustrated story of a client's life. The timelines were often used productively in subsequent individual sessions. This activity increased reality orientation and prompted self-reflection. Many times significant details emerged through this activity that did not come up in traditional talk therapy.

Inspired by: Similar activities seen at other treatment centers.

Timelines HANDOUT

TIMELINES

Think of your life story as a timeline. What are the important or meaningful events that have happened in your life? These can include events that are happy, sad, or painful to remember. You might include moving, births, deaths, other losses, school, work, pets, friends, first use of alcohol or other drugs, or anything large or small that stands out.

On the left, start with when and where you were born. On the right, at the end, list today's date and location. What happened in between? How did you get here? Include as many events as you wish.

I was born   **Today**

"Allow yourself to see what you
don't allow yourself to see."

Milton H. Erickson

Walk the Line

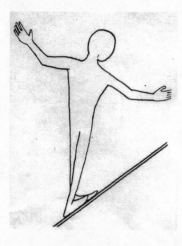

Location: Outdoors (an area where people can spread out)

Time: 30 minutes

Materials: A platform where the facilitator can be seen by the group (steps, picnic table, or chair)

Line on the ground with space on each side (use chalk or a string)

Walk the Line Handout (for facilitator)

Objectives

- To provide an opportunity to reflect upon different areas in life.
- To evaluate how these areas can enhance success or pose additional challenges to recovery.

Directions

1. Read aloud the following directions:

   The purpose of this activity is to provide an opportunity to reflect upon different areas in each of our lives and how these areas can enhance success or pose additional challenges to recovery. There are no right or wrong answers in this activity. It is a self-inventory of how things are for each one of us, here and now. If you are blessed with a lot of positive factors that help your recovery, use them well. If you are faced with a lot of challenges, be aware that you will need to work hard to overcome difficulties. Self-awareness is one of the things that helps you make wise decisions. Find pride in your own awareness and in your own ability to take positive strides, despite challenges.

2. Draw a line on a sidewalk or other flat area that everyone can stand next to in a single-file line.

3. Identify one side of the line as **Strengths** and the other side as a **Challenges**.

4. Read aloud one of the attributes from the Walk the Line Handout. Each time an attribute is called out, direct participants to take one step in the direction of strengths or challenges. It is up to each person to decide if something is a strength or a challenge for him or her. It may not be the same for everyone.

5. At the conclusion of this activity, have participants take inventory of their relative position of strengths or challenges. Encourage them to discuss what they have learned; some may notice that many share the same experiences.

Observations

This activity was done in beautiful weather on the basketball court as part of a series of outdoor activities. Twenty-seven group members participated, and the activity maintained full attention for longer than thirty minutes. The enthusiasm of the group was genuine and contagious. The spread on each side of the line was unexpectedly vast. Some women took giant steps to represent major strengths or challenges, and one woman took twenty-five steps to represent each of her grandchildren. Several took very large steps to represent their anger management challenges. A few women seemed to have setbacks each time they approached a position of strength. After going through the list, a large group had hit the fence on the strengths side, and a small group remained on the challenges side. One woman had never left the challenge side and was counseled afterward. She was aware, philosophical, and expressed that it showed what she already knew—she was going to have to work extra hard. Most of the participants expressed surprise at the way others shared similar struggles.

Inspired by: Johnny Cash's song and a popular children's party game.

Walk the Line HANDOUT

Attributes: Do you have a strength or a challenge?

Do you have a high school diploma?

Do you have family members that use alcohol or other drugs?

Do you have children to love?

Do you have job skills?

Do you have a home waiting for you?

Do you have health problems?

Is there food in your pantry?

Do you have a bank account?

Do you have money in the bank?

Do you have a car?

Do you have a driver's license?

Do you know your social security number?

Do you know where your social security card is?

Do you belong to a church?

Do you have a copy of your birth certificate?

Do you have a sponsor?

Do you have a sponsor who you have talked to in the last week?

Do you have a home group?

Do you have friends who don't use?

Have you been in recovery for thirty days?

Have you been in recovery for ten days?

Have you been in recovery for five days?

Do you think you might have anger management problems?

Do you know how to smile?

Do you believe in yourself?

Are you honest with yourself?

Are you loyal to yourself?

Do you have spirituality?

Do you have a role model?

Do you know where you want to be next month?

Can you picture yourself successful?

Are you worried about something?

Do you have dental problems?

Do you have clothes suitable for a job interview?

Have you written a good-bye letter to your addiction?

Have you done a good deed today?

Is your room clean?

Have you learned something about yourself today?

Have you completed your first step?

Have you created a relapse prevention plan?

Do you know your triggers?

Can you control your cravings?

Have you ever faced your cravings and successfully overcome them without using?

Have you written a letter to a friend or loved one within the last year?

Can you look in the mirror and feel good about what you see?

Have you taken a shower within the last twenty-four hours?

Do you smoke cigarettes?

Do you borrow or steal cigarettes to keep up the habit?

Have you told someone you love them within the last thirty days?

Have you done treatment work that wasn't required?

Have you cleaned up after someone else?

Have you done a chore without complaint?

Have you smelled a flower this week?

Have you done a morning meditation?

Have you given someone a compliment?

Have you had a good dream that you remember?

Have you been late to group?

Do you wake up in the morning feeling happy?

Do you cross talk in groups?

Do you look forward to tomorrow?

Have you set a good example for someone else this week?

Have you ever had a bad hair day?

Do you know how to have a good relationship with another person?

Is someone you care about in a gang?

Have you ever been in a gang?

Do you think you are over or under weight?

Have people told you that you are over or under weight?

Do you care about someone who has HIV or AIDS?

Did someone insult you and it hurt you?

Have you given someone a compliment?

Have you said "thank you" this week?

Walk a Mile in My Shoes

Location: Indoors (need tables or workspace)

Time: 90 minutes

Materials: Secondhand shoes of varioius styles (one shoe per person)

Paint (water-based or acrylic)

Large sheets of paper or cardboard (at least 12" × 18") or foamboard (one per person)

Glue or glue sticks

Scissors

Collage materials, sequins, jewel shapes, glitter, feathers

Optional: Speakers to play the song "Walk a Mile in My Shoes," originally performed by Joe South and The Believers, or similar songs

Objectives

- To encourage participants to tell their life story.
- To encourage unconditional self-acceptance.

Directions

1. Before the session, collect an assortment of used shoes—a variety of heels, flats, and athletic shoes based on the gender make-up of the group. They do not have to match or be wearable. Shoes can be purchased cheaply at garage sales, or secondhand stores might donate unusable pairs.

2. Have participants select one base to use as a display board and one shoe.

3. On the top of the paper, direct participants to write, *If you walk in my shoes . . .* followed by what others might not know about their lives or what others might not immediately see about their lives. Encourage participants to write about positive things as well as losses or struggles.

4. Instruct participants to paint or decorate their shoe and attach it with glue to the display board.

5. After everyone has finished, invite each participant to present his or her shoe and story to the group.

Observations

Women often prefer working with the high heels, and men can use athletic shoes. Female participants delighted in this activity and engaged in it immediately. It was an enjoyable way for them to approach telling their story. Those who found it difficult to share in traditional process groups viewed this activity as a safe way to start communicating with others.

Inspired by: A similar activity seen at the Metro Dallas Homeless Alliance, Dallas, Texas.

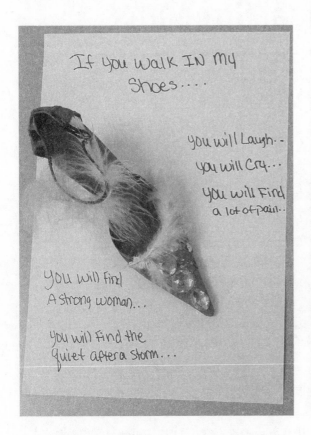

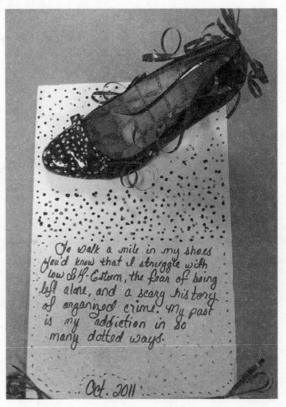

"If you walk in my shoes . . . you will laugh . . . you will cry . . . you will find a lot of pain . . . you will find a strong woman . . . you will find the quiet after a storm . . .

"To walk a mile in my shoes you'd know that I struggle with low self-esteem, the fear of being left alone, and a scary history of organized crime. My past is my addiction in so many dotted ways."

Self-Awareness: Individual Strengths and Areas for Growth

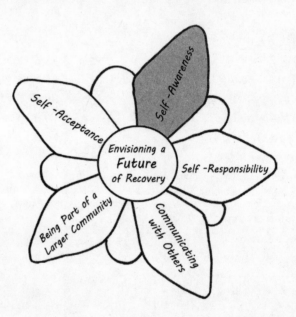

Activities in this section are targeted at increasing awareness of individual strengths. Rediscovery of existing abilities and learning new abilities reinforces the expectation that this process is cumulative and self-sustainable.

Abilities are highly individualistic, and these activities emphasize working together to find one's own strengths. Recovery groups provide safe and accepting opportunities for participants to explore simple skills and to reflect on where competencies are at the moment.

Roxanna: When working with large groups, there are always a few individuals who stand out as having special talent at a particular activity. Cultivating a group atmosphere of support for one another is one area I consider to be my own strength. I believe that while some proficiencies are special talents, much of what separates one group member from another is a combination of life experiences and learned skills.

Even acts as simple as cutting with scissors or knowing how to fold a piece of gift wrap do not come innately; they come from learning. By keeping the focus of our activities on a growth process, I don't hesitate to reveal my own limitations. My mother encouraged my sensitivity to and appreciation for the differences of others. By showing my personal, imperfect model of what it is to be human, I nourish a greater latitude of willingness to accept one's own limitations.

What has been most surprising is the frequent and many ways participants reveal talents. In working on one project, it is not unusual for the participants to take advantage of art supplies or flexible time to explore something within themselves. These spontaneous inspirations stimulate others to respond in positive ways. One woman who kept an empty cigarette box of found items shared it with us, and we adopted it into the "Strength Box" activity. Unexpected moments of discovery are truly the richest part of working with our clients.

Kay: I have observed that individuals in residential treatment for addiction or mental illness commonly do not know who they are anymore. They may have used substances or struggled with mental illness for so long they have forgotten what unique qualities define them as a person. It is affirming to help people find talents and aptitudes they thought were lost.

The "Diamante Poems" and "Haiku" poems and activities allow connected associations to emerge, and the resulting spontaneous creativity displayed is impressive. Focusing on positive past and present experiences, part of the "Gratitude Sheets" and "Positive Recollections" activities, help clients envision a positive future for themselves.

Box It Up

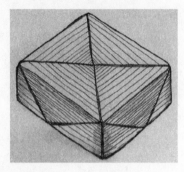

Location: Indoors

Time: 60 minutes

Materials: 8" × 8" paper squares (at least three sheets per person)

Scissors

Box It Up Handout (one per person)

Optional: Markers

Objectives

- To create an origami box for personal use.
- To self-identify ways in which the box can be used to support recovery.
- To provide a sense of accomplishment using the simple, yet exacting, nature of origami and improvement with practice.

Directions

1. Before the session, it may be useful to create a sample of each step of the box-making process, as well as a sample of a completed box.

2. Pass out the Box It Up Handout.

3. Have participants select three sheet of paper. As they follow the instructions, encourage them to fold paper carefully and to notice ways that improvement is seen with each successive attempt. If the box has a lid, it can be constructed by trimming the paper approximately ¼ inch on two sides. This will construct a box that is just small enough to slip snugly inside the first one.

4. Invite volunteers to share what they thought about the activity and what they might place in the box.

Observations

This activity was done with large groups. Approximately half of the participants were able to make a box with only these instructions and the model at the front of the room. The rest requested some individual help or reassurance. All but one participant constructed a box, and many participants constructed several in the time allowed. Those who had experience helped others who needed assistance. It should be stressed that the benefit in this activity is in the effort: the act of concentration and doing the folding movements. These benefits may be gained apart from the look of the finished product. There is no right or wrong outcome, and the emphasis should not be on whether a completed box looks nice. In the discussions that followed, there was enthusiastic and appropriate commentary regarding the creative manner in which the participants envisioned using the boxes in constructive ways, most of which were directly associated with success in recovery. The uses anticipated by participants included holding photos of children or other keepsakes. One client talked about symbolically putting her "past" in the box and leaving it there.

Inspired by: This origami project was inspired by a client who spontaneously constructed an origami box in an unrelated group.

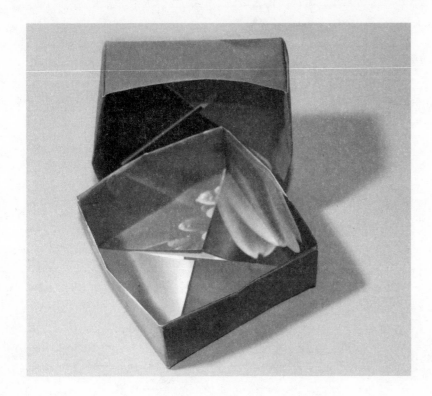

Box It Up HANDOUT

This activity requires two pieces of square paper.

The more exact your folds, the more artistic the box will appear.

With each fold, fold in one direction frontward, then backward, leaving a crease.

A legend is provided to help with the visual aids.

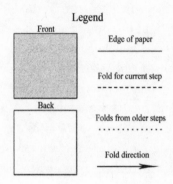

Legend

Front

Edge of paper

Fold for current step

Back

Folds from older steps

Fold direction

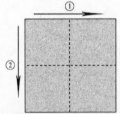

Step 1: Fold the paper left to right, crease and unfold.

Step 2: Fold the paper from top to bottom, crease and unfold.

Step 3: Turn the paper over.

Step 4: Fold each corner into the center, making a smaller square.

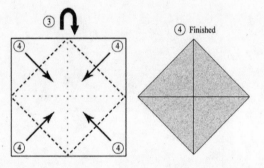

④ Finished

Step 5: Fold the outer edge to the center, crease, unfold. Repeat for the remaining three sides.

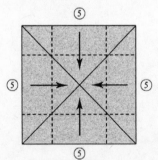

Step 6: Fully open two opposite sides of the square.

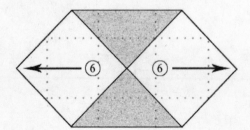

Step 7: Fold the two side walls so that they stand up straight.

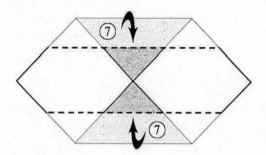

Step 8: Pinch the two side walls together on one end, They should almost touch.

Step 9: Fold the pointed edge over the wall created in Step 8. It should tuck together and finish the third wall.

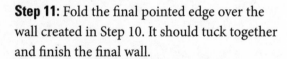

Step 10: Pinch the two sides together on the other end.

Step 11: Fold the final pointed edge over the wall created in Step 10. It should tuck together and finish the final wall.

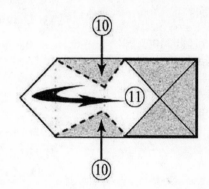

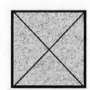

Finished

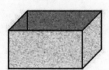

Congratulations, you created an origami box!

To make a lid, create a second box using slightly larger paper.

Brochure About Me

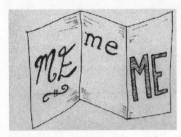

Location: Indoors

Time: 90 minutes

Materials: Plain sheets of 8.5" × 14" paper

Pens, markers, or colored pencils

Paper clips (one per person)

Optional: Collage or scrapbook paper

Objectives

- To encourage positive self-image and self-exploration.
- To help identify strengths within.
- To facilitate giving positive feedback to peers.

Directions

1. Before the session, place pens, paper clips, and art materials on each table or on a side table for participants to help themselves.
2. Distribute the Quiz About Me and have participants complete the quiz.
3. Ask participants to move to tables or a work area where they have room to spread out their materials.
4. Pass out the brochure directions—one per participant or table. Demonstrate folding the trifold, steps 1 and 2.
5. Review the remaining directions starting with step 3.
6. Pass out one piece of paper to participants and have them follow the directions.

Observations

The brochures were amazingly creative. Participants expressed feeling more emotionally positive after contemplating their strengths. Those with a weaker self-image found significant support and encouragement from the comments others wrote about them.

Inspired by: Adapted from similar activities done in school settings to reinforce self-esteem.

Brochure About Me HANDOUT

Brochure Directions

1. Take one sheet of paper. Fold into thirds, so you have a trifold brochure with three rectangular panels.

2. Unfold the paper you can see three panels.

3. On the three panels that will be the inside, write some or all of your completed sentences from the quiz.

4. Turn the paper over. This will be the outside of your brochure.

5. On the outside, put your name in the panel on the right (#3). Illustrate as desired.

6. Leave the left and center panels (#1 and #2) blank.

7. Fold over the panel on the right (#3), so that your name shows on the outside. Use a paper clip to keep the panel closed.

8. Turn the paper so the two blank panels are facing up.

9. Give the brochure to another person, inviting them to write a positive comment in one of the blank panels.

10. Pass the brochure to another person, then another, until both panels are full.

11. At the end, you will have a brochure that is filled with healthy comments from yourself on the inside and positive comments to you from others on the outside.

1	2	3

Brochure About Me HANDOUT

Quiz About Me

Complete these sentences with your own answers.
Use this information to put in your brochure.

My favorite color is _____

One of my favorite meals is _____

I love being sober because _____

_____

_____

My best feature is _____

My favorite activity for fun is _____

Something I am good at is _____

My proudest moment is _____

_____

_____

I rejoice in _____

_____

I believe in myself because _____

_____

_____

_____

My heart feels good when _____

_____

_____

I have faith in _____

_____

_____

If I were an animal, I would be a _____ because _____

_____

I would like to learn how to _____

It relaxes me when I _____

When I leave here, one coping skill I will use to stay sober is _____

_____

_____

Life will be better sober because _____

_____

_____

_____

_____

_____

_____

Claywork: Making Pinch Pots

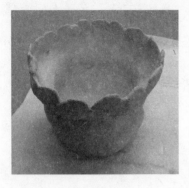

Location: Indoors

Time: 90–120 minutes

Materials: Air-dry clay

Wax paper

Forks, spoons, or other tools

Paper towels

Spray water bottles

Pieces of cardboard or foam board

Claywork Handout (one per person)

Optional: Acrylic paints

Objectives

- To provide a tactile, nonverbal activity.
- To provide a primal method of expression by rolling and manipulating clay.
- To use a focused task to stimulate touch and enhance self-awareness.

Directions

1. Before the session, buy or order clay in advance, sufficient for the number of participants. Air-dry or oven-bake clay are available from online art supply outlets. Twenty-five pounds of air-dry clay was enough for approximately twelve to fourteen participants. If you have not made a simple pinch pot before, practice before you do this with your group.

2. Ask everyone to wear old clothes to this activity.

3. Demonstrate how to make a pinch pot.

4. Pass out the Claywork Handout with detailed instructions.

5. Give everyone a piece of wax paper to work the clay on.

6. Hand each person a piece of clay, approximately the size of a tennis ball.

7. Tell participants to use forks, spoons, or other tools to create designs on the soft clay.

8. When clients are done, they can take the pots and let them dry for 24 to 48 hours.

9. If desired, tell participants their dried pots can be decorated with acrylic paints. Also the pots can be shellacked or decorated with glue, beads, shells, or other materials.

Observations

Many participants had not played with clay since elementary school, and several had never made a pot. The rolling and pinching of the thick clay was engaging and soothing. The density and texture of natural clay provides an intense physical experience that leads to a lasting finished product.

Inspired by: Pottery classes taken as a child.

Claywork HANDOUT

Making Pinch Pots

The technique used to make pinch pots is one of the oldest methods of claywork. Pinch pots, made from balls of clay into which fingers or thumbs are inserted to make the opening, may have been the very first pottery. Traditionally, women often made clay pots to put grain, food, and water in, such as Native American or Pueblo women living in the Southwest.

Directions

1. Begin by compressing your clay into a ball with your hands. Make a solid clay ball, about the size of a tennis ball.

2. Holding your ball in one hand, use your other thumb to push down, creating a well in the center of the ball. Make it deep but not so deep as to push through the bottom of the pot.

3. Using your thumb and index finger, pinch and press the clay upward with each movement of your fingers. Turn the ball of clay slowly in your hand as you pinch the sides. Try to keep the sides evenly thick.

4. Beginning at the bottom of your piece, work the clay upward forming the wall and size of your pot. Do this completely around the pot while pressing the clay slightly upward with each pinch or push of the clay. It is important to try and keep consistent movements while pinching or pressing.

5. Pinch your clay upward inside the pot until you come back where you started. Gently draw your top inward. Move your fingers up and begin a new row. Each time you have completed a circle around the inside of the pot, begin again on a new row until you have all of your clay pinched up.

6. Once you have reached the top, begin again at the bottom and work the wall upward again.

7. Gently tap your pot on a flat surface to form a flat bottom.

8. After you have finished pinching your pot, use your fingers to check for lumps, or too much bunched-up clay inside the pot. Using your fingers, smooth the outside surface, checking for lumps or undistributed clay.

9. If you wish, you can use a slightly smaller pinch pot to create a top for your pot. You can make a lid, or you can smooth the top into the bottom to make a taller pot.

10. Use a fork, spoon, stick, or other object to decorate your pot.

11. Place your pot on a piece of cardboard and let it air dry for 24 to 48 hours.

12. After drying, you can decorate your pot with acrylic paints, if desired.

Steps to Make a Pinch Pot

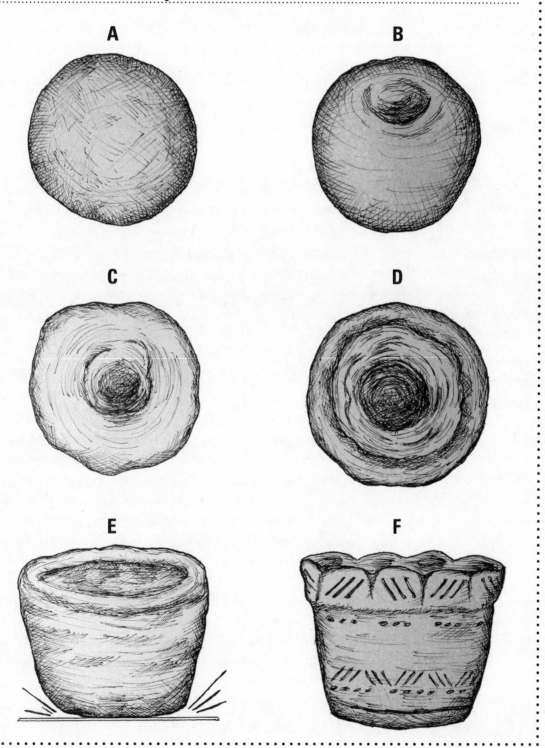

A

B

C

D

E

F

Counting Sheep

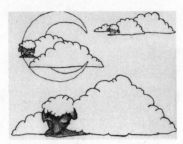

Location: Indoors

Time: 40 minutes

Materials: Bulletin board

Thumbtacks

Background paper for board

Counting Sheep Handout and Template (one per person)

Markers or crayons

Scissors

Objectives

- To increase awareness of sleep patterns.
- To encourage self-reflection of own problem-solving strategies.
- To give participants the opportunity to learn from others' problem-solving techniques.

Directions

1. Begin with general discussion regarding sleep hygiene.
2. Solicit tips from participants who have a technique for falling asleep.
3. Invite participation on group bulletin board to display successful strategies (naturalistic methods, not medications).
4. Offer Counting Sheep Template and art supplies to participants.
5. Encourage participation and learning from one another.
6. End with voluntary oral sharing of tips to the whole group.
7. Pass out the Tips for a Good Night's Sleep for further discussion.

Observations

Sheep templates were given to fifteen participants at the conclusion of a group in which the topic was sleep hygiene. The interactive portion had been done within the group; the bulletin board project was an optional component and available to the larger general population. Blank sheep remained available throughout the week, and the bulletin board evolved to fill the space. Participants reflected what had been discussed in cognitive groups and tapped into personal strategies for rest and relaxation. For more information, see the National Institute of Health website.

Inspired by: Difficulty sleeping is a common complaint from individuals in early recovery.

Counting Sheep TEMPLATE

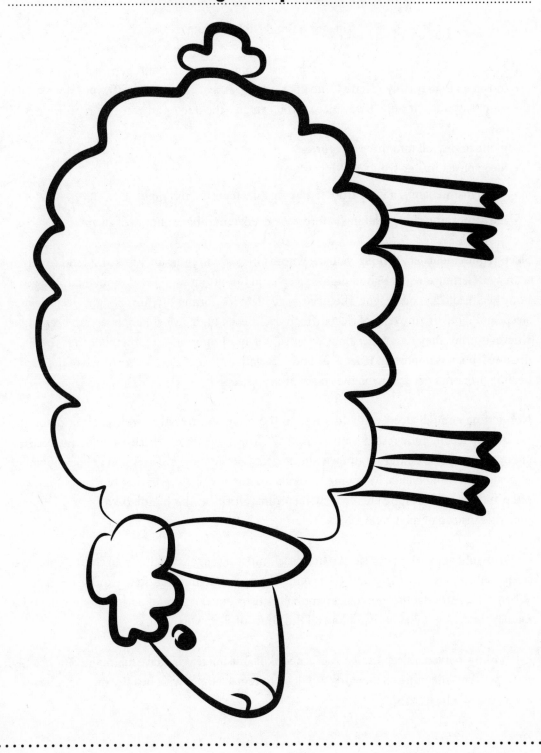

Counting Sheep HANDOUT

Tips for a Good Night's Sleep

Most adults need six to nine hours of sleep every night. Know what your personal requirements are and adapt to them. If you have difficulty sleeping, and need to speak with your doctor, take the time to evaluate it fully in advance so you can give the doctor an accurate report.

Sleep difficulties fall into three categories:

- Sleep onset, having trouble falling asleep

- Sleep maintenance, having trouble staying asleep for the full night

- Early morning rising, waking before your needed number of hours of sleep

Sleep requirements are lifelong, but sleep needs increase in times of stress and tend to lessen with age. Getting a regular good night's sleep is an important ingredient to maintaining good body health and a good weight. The sleep cycle includes normal rhythms of light sleep, deeper sleep, and rapid eye movement sleep, which occur each night. Most people dream each night whether or not they remember their dreams. It is not important to remember that you have dreamed, but it is important to let your body reach that stage of deep sleep. Much of the body's healing processes occur during the stages of deep sleep.

Not getting enough sleep will add stress to the body and interfere with healing potential. Waking up feeling fully rested is nice but not a clear indicator of whether or not one has had enough sleep. Establishing a routine bedtime and wake-up time are useful in the development of healthy sleeping habits. Many medications interfere with sleep cycles, but adaptation can often be achieved despite this. Most sleep difficulties can be handled with simple home remedies instead of medications.

If you are unhappy with your sleep patterns, eliminating sugar, caffeine, tobacco, alcohol, and sleep medications is a simple way to let your own natural rhythms begin to express themselves. When trying to establish good sleeping habits, it is better to wake up in the morning at a regular time even if you have not had all the hours of sleep you want.

Establishing personal sleep habits is a learned skill. The longer you have maintained unhealthy sleep patterns, the more challenging it will be to replace them with healthy ones, but healthy habits can still be learned.

The following tips may be useful to develop healthy sleep routines:

- It is generally better to avoid naps, and try again the next night.

- Taking naps after a sleepless night interferes with the development of good sleep.

- Do not make it a habit of spending time in bed for reading, watching TV, or other awake-time activities. Train yourself to associate your bed with sleeping.

- Know your best sleep hours and respect them.

- Limit stimulating activities, including exercise or computer work, near bedtime.

- Avoid caffeine, chocolate, tobacco, alcohol, and other drugs.

- Manage environmental conditions, including temperature, sounds, and lighting, to your own preferences that will favor your ability to sleep comfortably.

- Establish nightly rituals to cue your body that sleep is approaching, such as teeth brushing, dimming lights, or putting on your pajamas.

- Old-fashioned remedies, such as chamomile tea, a teaspoon of honey, or a warm glass of milk, may have a physical basis to enhance relaxation.

- A warm bath can relax muscles and stimulate internal temperature changes that can help encourage sleep.

- Choose bedding, such as a pillow and blanket, that support feelings of safety and comfort. Different people prefer different fabrics.

- Learn a few relaxation techniques, such as restful breathing, mindful moments, sensory exploration, or progressive relaxation, to invite sleep.

- If sleep does not come within half an hour of settling into bed, it may be useful to get up and repeat the going-to-bed ritual, without going on to other activities.

- Even if you are not asleep, stay in bed during your sleep hours.

- If are awake, lying still with your eyes closed can supply healing rest.

- A trip to the bathroom need not interfere with a good night's rest.

- When you awaken in the morning, take a few moments to notice the feeling of being very close to sleep and enjoy that sensation.

- Exposure to daylight is an effective way to stimulate the body to wake up.

- Get some physical exercise during the daytime.

Healthy sleep habits are easier to maintain than to establish. Commit yourself to working on finding what works for you, then keep it up.

Cut Me In

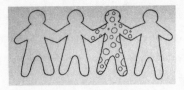

Location: Indoors

Time: 40 minutes

Materials: Scissors

Variety of colored papers (standard or legal size)

Crayons, colored pencils, or markers

Paper plates

Tape or glue

Objectives

- To reflect on the chains of effect we have on people around us.

- To envision representations of support systems in their lives.

Directions

1. Pass out paper to all participants.

2. Demonstrate the folding and cutting techniques.

   A. Fold paper vertically. Fold again on the same axis so the paper is now four layers and shaped like a tall rectangle.

   B. Fold paper horizontally. This creates the mid-line for the paper figure.

   C. On the top half of the paper, cut a head and two arms. To make the paper figures connect, the arms need to extend pass the edge of the folded sheet. Do not make any cuts in the bottom half.

   D. Unfold and show the four figures holding hands.

   E. Working on individual figures within the chain, cut out pant legs or skirts as desired.

3. Have participants create their figure chain. Tell them that the figures can represent immediate family or various support people. Also the paper figures can be used to illustrate various factors, such as substance use within families. To add more figures, two chains can be taped or glued together.

4. Have the participants use the paper plates to collect the scraps of paper, simplifying cleanup.

5. Encourage participants to decorate the figures as desired.

Observations

A group of twenty-seven enthusiastically embraced this activity, decorating the cutouts lavishly. Several showed themselves holding hands with children or Alcoholics Anonymous sponsors. One showed herself in the center of a chain of three figures and described herself as being simultaneously pulled in opposite directions by addiction and recovery. Creative expression was welcomed and several showed innovative adaptations to the activity, constructing butterflies, baby chickens, and robots. Several clients also decorated the paper plates. One made a chain long enough to represent everyone in the facility. While markers, colored-paper trimmings, and crayons were all available for use, crayons were selected most frequently.

Inspired by: Old-fashioned paper doll play and the expressed wishes by women who had never learned the technique of creating them.

Diamante Poems

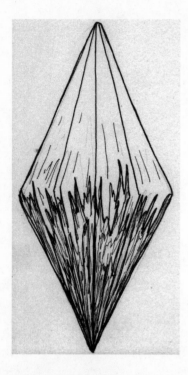

Location: Indoors

Time: 60 minutes

Materials: Lists of adjectives and verbs (can be optional, depending on literacy of group)

Diamante Poems Handout

Diamante Poems Template

Decorative supplies

Construction paper

Sample poem

Objectives

- To encourage exploration, discovery, and group work as a means for self-reflection and expression.

Directions

1. Read sample aloud. Create your own or use one of the provided samples.

2. Discuss how diamante poems transition from the beginning to end. Explain that these are seven-line poems in which the words form a diamond shape, and two ideas or opposite concepts are contrasted. They verbally illustrate the shift that occurs in the process of moving from one opposite to another.

3. As a group, generate a few opposite constructs that can be used for the poems.

4. Guide the group to create the first diamante poem as a team.

5. Read aloud the group's diamante poem.

6. Direct participants to construct their own diamante poem showing their transition from substance use to recovery using the Diamante Poems Handout and Template.

7. Invite participants to read aloud their completed poems.

8. Encourage participants who finish early to transfer their poems to construction paper and decorate as desired.

Observations

This activity was done on three occasions with six, eight, and ten participants. Depending on the education and literacy level of your population, instructional needs will vary. The activity went smoothly when a template was used with the type of word needed for each line, and another template with blank spaces to write the words on. Some participants may have difficulty with instructions, but group work proved effective in clarifying expectations and stimulating interest. When particiapants used vocal volume to emphasize the contrast, this provided clarification. Everyone chose to transfer their poems to colored construction paper and decorate.

Inspired by: There are numerous examples of this technique in manuals and online curricula for school teachers. This activity was adapted from these sources.

These poems were written in groups:

TIRED
Ragged Groggy
Sleeping Snoring Resting
Bed Pillow Alarm Daylight
Yawning Stretching Looking
Refreshed Bright
AWAKE

SEED
Tiny Fragile
Growing, Changing, Rooting
Leaf Sprig Branch Wood
Spreading Shading Supporting
Tall Branches
TREE

A finished individual poem that reads:

DRUNK
intoxicated disturbing
self-delusion self-pity self-seeking
ill ashamed balanced happy
generous self-sacrificing hopeful
willingness honesty
SOBER

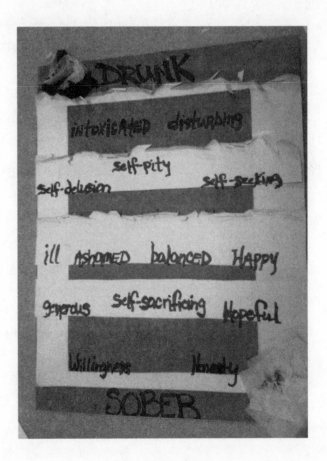

Diamante Poems HANDOUT

Instructions

Start by filling in a pair of ideas: beginning idea and ending idea.

The ideas should be opposites or very different from each other.

Example: hot/cold or asleep/awake.

The activity makes a transformation from whatever you choose as a beginning idea to the ending idea.

1. Beginning idea: Substance Use/Abuse.

2. Two words that describe (adjective) the beginning idea.

3. Three -*ing* words (verbs) that describe activities related to the beginning idea.

4. Two word pictures (nouns) that relate to the beginning idea.
   Two word pictures that relate to the ending idea.

5. Three -*ing* words (verbs) that describe activities relating to ending idea.

6. Two words that describe (adjectives) the ending idea.

7. Ending idea: RECOVERY.

FORMAT: WHAT TO PUT ON EACH LINE
1. BEGINNING IDEA

2. DESCRIBE   DESCRIBE

(two words describing beginning idea)

3. --------ING   ------ING   ------ING

(action words describing beginning idea)

4. PICTURE   PICTURE   PICTURE   PICTURE

(two nouns describing beginning idea)   (two nouns describing ending idea)

5. --------ING   ------ING   ------ING

(action words describing ending idea)

6. DESCRIBE   DESCRIBE

(two words describing ending idea)

7. ENDING IDEA

Diamante Poems TEMPLATE

TITLE
AUTHOR

1. _____

2. _____ _____

3. _____ _____ _____

4. _____ _____ _____ _____

5. _____ _____ _____

6. _____ _____

7. _____

Diamante Poems TEMPLATE

TITLE
AUTHOR

1. _____

2. _____ _____

3. _____ _____ _____

4. _____ _____ _____ _____

5. _____ _____ _____

6. _____ _____

7. _____

ACTION WORDS FOR POEMS: VERBS

TRY	CONTEMPLATE	SMELL	WRITE
RUN	CONSIDER	STAND	DRAW
WALK	WONDER	SQUEEZE	WORK
CRAWL	QUESTION	BREATHE	REMEMBER
GO	STRUGGLE	LOVE	PRETEND
STOP	LIVE	ADORE	DREAM
REACH	ENJOY	LIKE	DESCRIBE
CARRY	EAT	WANT	ACCOMPLISH
PICK UP	ABSORB	CLOSE	FINISH
IMAGINE	TRY	OPEN	WIN
THINK	ATTEMPT	PEEK	REACH
ENVISION	THROW	LOOK	FIND
TALK	TOSS	SEE	PLAN
ASK	DISPLAY	SING	EXPLORE
BEG	CRY	SHARE	PAINT
DEMAND	SHOUT	STORE	SIT
PRAY	YELL	SIGN	
THINK	WHISPER	REST	
HOPE	STRETCH	WORK	

DESCRIPTIVE WORDS FOR POEMS: ADJECTIVES

PRETTY	THIN	COLD-HEARTED	PEACEFUL
KIND	THICK	SNEAKY	POWERFUL
BEAUTIFUL	OLD	JOYFUL	DISMAL
LOVELY	NEW	GIGGLY	FUNNY
HURRIED	YOUNG	SAD	DUMB
STRESSED	BUBBLY	MISERABLE	STUPID
ENERGETIC	SLEEPY	FRIGHTFUL	AMAZING
GENEROUS	DROWSY	FRIGHTENING	FANTASTIC
HELPFUL	LIVELY	SCARY	AWESOME
WORRIED	UGLY	HORRIFYING	GREAT
QUIET	WISE	MORTIFYING	COOL
SMART	THOUGHTFUL	DREADFUL	MIRACULOUS
GRACEFUL	CONSIDERATE	HOT	WONDERFUL
SMOOTH	CARING	FINE	OUTSTANDING
SWEET	MINDFUL	HAPPY	
USUAL	MINDLESS	MERRY	
EXTRAORDINARY	HEARTLESS	GRACEFUL	

Emotions in Two Colors

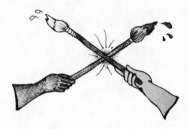

Objectives

- To explore feelings and emotions in a safe and symbolic way.

- To visibly explore the balance and interplay of strong feelings.

- To offer a sense of opportunity to move beyond past difficulties.

Directions

1. Begin with an overview of the purpose of the activity, not as an art project but as a way of expressing emotions that are hard to put into words.

2. Have a group discussion regarding various emotions. Consider those that are positive (happy, joy, energized, comfortable, laughter, feeling strong) and those that are negative (sad, embarrassed, angry, confused, bored, victimized, mad). Refer to the Feelings Words Handout in the Appendix.

3. Direct participants to choose three colors to work with. They should use a background color representing life, one color representing a positive emotion, and another color representing a negative emotion.

4. Instruct participants to tear positive and negative emotion papers into shapes to illustrate how the two emotions affect each other.

5. Encourage volunteers to show their work to the group and explain what their illustration means.

Location: Indoors

Time: 45 Minutes

Materials: Construction paper

Glue or glue sticks

Pens

Lined paper

Optional: Finger paints (instead of colored paper)

Feeling Words Handout page 342

Observations

This activity was done one time with torn, colored construction paper and a group of twelve, and a second time using finger paints with a group of twenty-seven. On both occasions it was challenging when offering choices of colors to enforce that the activity was designed for only a few colors. On both occasions some deep meaningful discussions ensued. About 25 percent of the participants wanted to share their stories, and others preferred to not put them into words. Most of the participants chose to keep their final products for personal display in their dorm rooms.

Inspired by: A project seen at a domestic violence shelter.

Feeling Boards

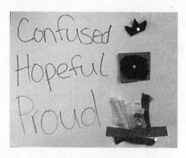

Location: Indoors

Time: 60–90 minutes

Materials: White cardstock (about 14" × 22"; one per person)

3" × 3" pieces of scrap fabric or other material (a variety of textures and may include velvet, felt, corduroy, burlap, sandpaper, vinyl, bubble wrap, netting)

Several bags for the fabric pieces

Round-headed brad fasteners (10 per person)

Markers or colored pencils

Scissors

Optional: List of Feeling Words (See Appendix.)

Objectives
- To have participants identify internal emotions using tactile sensation.

Directions

1. Before the session begins, prepare the following:

   A. Cut a variety of textured fabric or other collected materials in 3" × 3" pieces. These may be remnant fabric or other materials that have pronounced composition, such as sandpaper, shower curtain, shiny or textured paint chip samples, thin sponge, or bubble wrap.

   B. Make sure there are 10 pieces for each participant.

   C. Combine the pieces in several bags so people can reach in without seeing the contents.

   D. Make copies of the list of feeling words, if desired. Be sure to include both positive and negative emotions.

2. Ask participants to choose a piece of cardstock and write down some feelings or emotions they have currently or they identify with. If they cannot think of what they want to say, they can choose from the list of feeling words. Tell participants to leave space between each written emotion for one fabric piece. Suggest using three rows of three, making a total of nine, but allow participants to be creative. Cardstock may be folded over to make a book with a decorated cover.

3. Instruct participants to put their hands in a bag and choose a piece of material that feels like each emotion they wrote down, using only the touch of their hands, not eyesight.

4. Have participants attach each piece of fabric to the cardstock with metal brad fasteners.

5. Direct participants to decorate as desired.

6. Encourage participants to share their feeling board with the group, explaining why they chose each particular piece of material.

Observations

People who use alcohol and other drugs tend to numb their emotions, either intentionally or as a by-product of the drinking and drugging. In early recovery, emotions are often overwhelming, and it may be difficult to sort out what exactly one is feeling. Just asking someone, "So how do you feel today?", can be bewildering. This activity encourages clients to sort out and identify their emotions using tactile sensations instead of the usual words.

This activity was done in a large group of forty-five, but would be ideal for a smaller group. Participants embraced the idea quickly and came up with a variety of thoughtful creations. Those who had challenges with verbal expression found this activity to be very accessible. One client began the group with an angry, verbal altercation with another client. At the end of the activity, this client said that she felt much better and, using her feeling board, she expressed her moods in an insightful manner. Another client chose a piece of t-shirt material to represent gratitude because, as she explained, when she was homeless and had nothing she was grateful for a t-shirt.

Many participants looked at the fabric pieces as well as touched them to make their choices, which worked well. In a smaller group, it would be easier to limit the participants to only using the sense of touch.

Several participants commented spontaneously on how much they enjoyed this activity and how helpful it was for them.

Inspired by: Discussion with some of the women in recovery about how much comfort they felt when they were reminded of the softness of baby blankets or old clothes that they had worn. Thanks also to an activity experienced at the Betty Ford Center in Rancho Mirage, CA, for the idea for the Feeling Words.

Gratitude Sheets

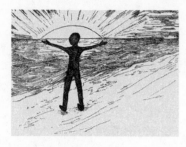

Location: Indoors

Time: 45–60 minutes (depending on group size)

Materials: Gratitude Sheets Handout

Objectives

- To promote a more positive way of thinking.
- To encourage a more positive spiritual state.
- To change "stinkin' thinkin'" into something more positive.

Directions

1. Before the session, familiarize yourself with the concept of resentment and gratitude in recovery.

2. Facilitate a discussion about resentment and gratitude. Explain that some people who work in recovery believe there should be three times the gratitude for every resentment. Ask the group to define the word *gratitude* and solicit reasons we might benefit from a more positive outlook for the present and the future.

3. Pass out the Moments of Gratitude Handout—you may wish to use another graphic depending on your audience.

4. Allow everyone to spend a few minutes writing at least five things they are grateful for today. These can be very small ideas or significant things.

5. Ask for volunteers to read aloud their moments of gratitude.

Observations

This activity was done many times on a Sunday morning when residents of the treatment center were feeling a little discontent and restless. It always refocused the participants on a more positive line of thought. As people shared their moments of gratitude with others, there was always laughter, and sometimes tears, and everyone left feeling more optimistic.

Inspired by: An activity done by Sandy G., long time counselor at Nexus Recovery Center in Dallas, Texas.

Gratitude Sheets HANDOUT

My Moments of Gratitude

_____

_____

_____

_____

_____

_____

_____

_____

_____

_____

_____

_____

_____

_____

_____

_____

_____

Haiku

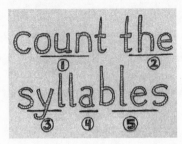

Location: Indoors

Time: 45 minutes

Materials: Haiku Handout (one per person)

Pens

Writing paper

Objectives

- To explore one's experience in recovery using a simple word art form.

- To explore the universality of experiencing and overcoming individual challenges.

Directions

1. Pass out the Haiku Handout. Ask participants to choose a single word or short phrase that will serve as a topic, such as *happy*.

2. Instruct participants to make a list of about a dozen words they associate with that topic.

3. Have participants count how many syllables are in each of the words they have listed, for example:
   Happy (2), Play (1), Smiling (2), Toys (1), Smile (1), Love (1), Run (1), Memories (3), Children (2), Today (2), Laughter (2), Everywhere (3), Fun (1), Giving (2).

4. Have participants arrange words into the three lines using the number of syllables (5-7-5).
   First line needs five syllables.
   Second line needs seven syllables.
   Third line needs five syllables.

5. Encourage participants to read silently and rearrange the words until the flow of the sounds and images becomes beautiful. Example:

Happy
Happy, Fun, Smiling
Children, Running, Laughter, Joy
Give, Love, Everywhere

Observations

This activity was done in a large group with active interest and engagement. A number of the participants had trouble counting out the syllables but remained interested despite this stumbling block. Some samples were offered from recovery websites to start off the participants. About half wrote about their recovery, while the remainder wrote about families or memories. All participants offered positive feedback, and several decorated their work. Even if a participant has trouble counting syllables (as in the poem "Sobriety" below), the outcome can still be powerful.

Inspired by: Elementary and middle school language exercises.

The following poems were written by group members.

Time
Me, getting older.
Not wiser, just drunk, help me.
Here now, recovery, today.

Lonely
Quiet Sad Hopeless
Empty Darkness One Unhappy
Needing Recovery

Daughters
Daughters Loving Fun
Joyful Beautiful Giving
Good Talented Moms

Sobriety
Sanity Begins
Fulfilled and Completed by Peace
Acceptance Reigns Whole

Haiku HANDOUT

Name _____

1. TOPIC _____

2. WORD LIST—Count the number of syllables in each word.

3. YOUR HAIKU—Write on the lines below.

1st LINE (5) _____ _____ _____ _____ _____

2nd LINE (7) _____ _____ _____ _____ _____ _____ _____

3rd LINE (5) _____ _____ _____ _____ _____

"Small moments of connection, often unexpectedly, can be the most gratifying."

KAY COLBERT

Memory Game

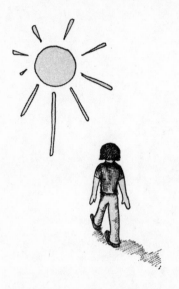

Location: Indoors

Time: 60–90 minutes

Materials: Writing supplies

Objectives

- To teach a way to learn or memorize new information.
- To help rebuild lost cognitive abilities through memory exercises.

Directions

1. Before the session, it is advised to practice this activity in advance, as it is more complex than most.

2. Begin with an orientation to the peg memory technique, which is learning to associate a list of items with easy-to-remember rhyming words. An effective opening to this activity is to read a shopping list of ten items and then ask individuals to write about what they remember. Typically about five or six items are remembered.

3. To introduce the peg memory technique, read a different shopping list, this time associating each item on the list with a peg anchor. Ask how many items participants can remember. Typically, the number increases dramatically. Read aloud the following explanation of how to use peg anchors.

   For each number, one through ten, a rhyming "anchor" or peg word is selected. Common ones are: One Sun, Two Shoe, Three Tree, Four Door, Five Sky Dive, Six Sticks, Seven Heaven, Eight Plate, Nine Vine, and Ten Hen. Once the anchor words are selected, I will read the shopping list, pausing to generate a visual image of the item on the shopping list in connection with the anchor word. The more fanciful or ridiculous the image the more powerful my recollection is likely to be. For example, the first two items on the shopping list, might be "ketchup" and "mustard." Using the previously named anchor words, my first image could be a bottle of ketchup in a bathing suit trying to get a sun tan. The second image could be mustard filling a shoe and spilling out over the top. Sequentially, I will go through each of the items on the shopping list, connecting the list items with the anchor words.

Observations

A mnemonic is an activity or technique to help with memory retention. It is thought that mnemonics use information already stored in our long-term memory to aid in learning new information. Often mnemonics involve auditory methods but can also include visual or kinesthetic methods. It may also be used to memorize any sequential list or strings of numbers, such as a phone number.

This activity was done both as a group project and as an individual project. Most seemed to enjoy the activity in both contexts. In a ninety-minute timeframe, it was attempted as a technique to remember the Twelve Steps. In this case, several participants complained that they already knew the Twelve Steps and did not need a technique to remember them. Others attempted to participate and found the application too complex. A small, self-selected group and constructed the poem below using the basic concepts.

Inspired by: Healthcare techniques to work with individuals with memory loss.

Example of a group composition to anchor the concept of the Twelve Steps

> It began on day ONE
> My horrible FUN
> Had blocked the SUN
> I looked up,
> TWO BLUE birds FLEW
> Tweeting: HE, not YOU
> THREE Words to God
> "Please help ME"
> I want to be FREE
> It's not like BEFORE
> I'll go through that DOOR
> I'll look inside and face what makes me SORE

I can still be ALIVE
Reach out: fingers FIVE, touch a hand to SURVIVE
"Get ready CHICKS
God can clean up the SICK"
I humbly ask Him for step SEVEN
"Cleanse me, get me ready for HEAVEN
Look at my PLATE,
All those I ATE
Undo that great WEIGHT
AGAIN and AGAIN
Dress me in NINE
I drop each a LINE
and confess: "My Bad, don't you PINE"
ON count of TEN
I make my AMENDS
Step ELEVEN,
Pray to HEAVEN
"God, Make me a better WOMAN"
Clock strikes TWELVE
More work on the SHELVES
Keep working through the dark to the sun,
Until all is DONE

Example of an "individual" composition

One Day I Looked to the Sun and Felt Powerless.

Today, It Blew My Mind, Blue can bring Sanity

See the three Father, Son, Holy Sprit

He awaits my decision to open the door For Discovery of what's within me.

Dive in Five fingers hand and hand

Ready for God to take the Sicks from within. Fix me.

Seventh heven pray he remove my shortcomings

Step thru the gate clean up what we are

nine plant a vine a garden of amends to give to my friends.

Ten minutes a day continue to grow taking notes with the den

Eleven heven on earth His will thur me

Twelve Dwell into the trenches to those in need.

Mirror Box

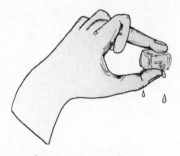

Location: Indoors or Outdoors

Time: 5 minutes per person (approximately)

Materials: 1 mirror box (12" × 12" mirrored tile, approximately 12" square box, duct tape)

Three or more items for exploration (Cold: ice or a frozen water bottle; Texture: something soft or bristly; Shapes: A rock or a bowl of beans)

A table at comfortable height to rest one's hands on while seated

Objectives

- To encourage the exploration of sensory malleability.

- To enhance the participants' belief in their own capacity for change through an perceived sensory response.

Directions

1. Before the session, try out the box prior to using it. To construct the mirror box, tuck the lid into the box and stand it on its side with the opening toward you. Attach the mirror to the exterior of the box (right or left side) using duct tape.

2. Demonstrates the desired positioning of the box. The mirror box should sit on the table with the opening facing the participant and the mirror just lateral of midline and tilted slightly toward the participant.

3. Position the first participant and the box to create the illusion of "seeing" both hands. With one hand resting on the table in front of the mirror, ask the participant to place the opposite hand into the box, generating the illusion that both the right and the left hands are visible. In fact, what is seen is one hand and its mirror image, while the opposite hand is concealed in the box.

4. Encourage the participant to let the unseen hand remain at rest and to move his or her visible hand while imagining the feeling occurring in both hands.

5. After a short interval of finger movement, provide the participant with an object from either the texture or shape category to invite the feeling within his or her exterior hand, moving the feeling to the hidden hand.

6. Encourage the participant to explore the sensations using three sequential items. When cold is used, encourage the feeling of coolness to migrate into the unseen hand.

7. Allow each participant a few minutes to explore his or her reactions.

8. Reinforce that unusual and transformative sensations come easier to some individual than others and a response is not

predictive of success in recovery. The purpose of the activity is only to encourage self-awareness and to discover a way that the body can learn to adapt.

Observations

A small group, up to eight participants, can engage in this activity because it is too individualistic to be useful in a larger group.

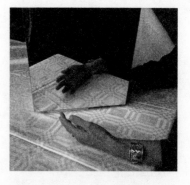

Example with right hand concealed in the box and left hand reflected in the mirror.

The cost of the construction was less than five dollars. Mirrored tiles are available in local hardware stores for two dollars. The box was obtained free of charge from a postal center. It took only a few minutes to construct.

This activity was performed several times with informal groups of volunteer participants in a variety of settings. It was tried with about twenty-five volunteers in a recovery setting as an individual free-time activity, not presented as a group. The experiences seemed to be more effective when the exploratory item was in the visible hand not the hidden hand. Overall, cold seemed to evoke the most reliable transfer of sensation but the response to texture, temperature, or shape seemed to be individualistic. In most cases, the unexpected sensations arising within the uninvolved limb was surprising and interpreted by the participant as evidence of learning to change. Often the sensation was rapid and dramatic, and the participants made powerful expressions of surprise and awe. In some cases, the response was slower causing the participant to work at opening his or her mind. A small minority could not engage in the sensation transformation. Overall, those who chose to participant consistently expressed appreciation and amazement with the experience.

Inspired by: The work of neuroscientist Vilayanur Ramachandran, director of the Center for Brain and Cognition at UCSD, and particularly his work on alleviation of phantom limb pain. Dr. Ramachandran developed a box which is somewhat more complex and uses two mirrors. His research has been of major influence in the alleviation of discomfort that often follows amputation. Similar mirror arrangements are used for rehabilitation from strokes.

Picture of Addiction and Recovery

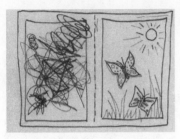

Location: Indoors

Time: 90 minutes

Materials: 9" × 12" paper

Colored paper

Markers

Scissors

Crayons

Glue

Optional: Magazines for collage

Objectives

- To engage a longer timeframe in personal reflection, going beyond the moment and into a larger awareness of one's life.

- To examine personal circumstances of substance abuse and recovery.

- To identify a transition from one lifestyle to healthier one.

Directions

1. Explain the activity and the purpose. Participants will illustrate the story of their addiction on the left side of a piece of paper. On the right side, they will illustrate what their recovery might look like.

2. Ask participants to select a piece of paper and fold it down the middle. Guide them to look at each side individually as well as the whole paper as a continuum.

3. Encourage free and honest expression.

4. As individuals conclude their work, facilitate a discussion and presentation to the larger group.

Observations

This activity was done a number of times in various sized groups. This seems to work well for groups of mixed ability, as few have difficulty starting with the troublesome expression of their addiction. Several of the participants became stalled at trying to envision a future of recovery. Being able to express uncertainty in this medium was reported to be extremely helpful. While the participants relaxed and enjoyed using magazines as collage materials, generally participants get more out of conceptualizing their own work with original drawings. Magazines can easily become a distraction from the focus of the project at hand. Repeatedly, participants showed chaotic and confusing images associated with addiction and loss. Some had associations of elements that they enjoyed, such as parties and high heels. The recovery side of the pictures tended to be either serene, sometimes expressions of tranquil lives of hope and peace, or an empty question of uncertainty. The process of making the picture increased self-awareness, was therapeutic, and elicited details that had not emerged in traditional narrative therapy. Whatever the participant showed provided fertile ground for discussion and support.

Inspired by: Collage work that participants did in free art times. Similar projects done in various treatment programs.

Positive Recollections

Location: Indoors

Time: 45–60 minutes

Materials: Positive Recollections Handout (one per person)

Pens

Objectives

- To promote a positive past orientation.
- To be successful in managing alcohol dependency than those with a more negative focus on the past.

Directions

1. Introduce the topic: Researchers found that alcoholics who focus on positive experiences in their past may be more successful in managing their addiction than those who had a more negative focus on the past. Also, discuss these other points from the study:

   A. Viewing past experiences more positively may aid recovery.

   B. People who were only focused on the here and now tended to experience stronger compulsions to drink alcohol.

   C. High levels of spiritualty (for example, finding purpose and meaning in life, the Twelve Step approach) were also found to be a protective factor in helping recovering alcoholics stay sober and manage the anxiety associated with addiction and withdrawal.

2. Distribute Positive Recollections Handout.

3. Ask each group member to write down a minimum of three positive things they remember from the recent or the distant past.

4. When everyone is done, invite people to read aloud what they have written.

Observations

This activity was done successfully multiple times. As the recollections were shared aloud, peers laughed or wept and truly appeared to empathize with other's memories.

Inspired by: The research study, "Living in the present: Time perspective and spirituality as predictors of sobriety and anxiety in recovering alcoholics," presented April 16, 2010, at the British Psychological Society by Sarah Davies and Gail Kinman of the University of Bedfordshire.

Positive Recollections HANDOUT

I Remember When . . .

_____

_____

_____

_____

_____

_____

_____

_____

_____

_____

_____

_____

_____

_____

Strength Boxes

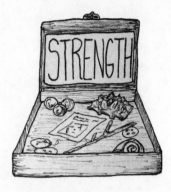

Location: Indoors or Outdoors (best with access to both)

Time: 60 minutes

Materials: Small boxes (one per person)

An assortment of random materials (tokens, buttons, safety pins, beads, marbles, or other small objects)

Art supplies

Sample strength box

Objectives

- To encourage thinking creatively about seeking support for ongoing recovery.

- To create a box filled with symbolic items that give a sense of strength for maintaining recovery.

Directions

1. Before the session, collect boxes and random symbolic items, which can be recycled from home. Also prepare a sample box to show participants.

2. Explain to the participants that small objects can serve as reminders to keep an individual resolute in recovery, and the objects can be symbolic or have meaning.

3. Show the group a sample box containing various natural objects, items, or images and provide sample explanations of how this can offer strength in a time of weakness.

4. Invite participants to select a box that "seems right" and to decorate it in their own style.

5. Once the box is decorated, direct participants to seek materials from those brought in, from their own resources, or collected from outdoors to use as contents for their strength box.

6. After 45 minutes, invite participants to show the group one or more items related to their box and to tell how it will help maintain recovery.

Observations

The facilitator brought an assortment of small boxes recycled from the household. Most of the boxes were about the size of a can of sardines. Additionally, a varied assortment of buttons, paper clips, clothespins, and other nominal objects were made available to supplement the participants' outdoor search in which they collected flowers, small stones, acorns, pieces of tree bark, and other items from nature. A group of more than forty women were invited to participate as a voluntary option to other activities. All forty chose participation and became actively engaged. Individuals responded with a vast array of creative responses. One found her own shoebox and filled it with flowers, then described the flowers as the beauty of being sober. One included images of the dawn and dusk. One carefully chose a stone which she then identified as her addiction and dramatically discarded it before the group. Another selected a plain box and filled it with damaged pieces of paper representing her life. She then selected items that represented the reparation process and noted how she is in a healing process. Several found photographs of family members to insert in their boxes.

The discussion portion was voluntary, and the majority of the participants expressed creative, heartfelt, and emotional responses to the activity. Many became tearful as they described the depth of meaning associated with symbols within their strength box. This activity enhanced effective and authentic expressive communication.

Inspired by: A client who collected bits of paper and other resources that she kept in an empty cigarette box she called her strength box. It had helped her in times of weakness.

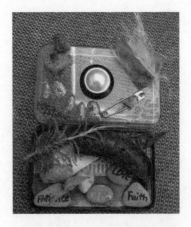

This box was filled with symbols for faith, love, and patience, as well as a note to self to be opened later.

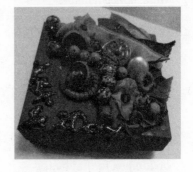

The cover of one box was collaged with acorns, dried mesquite pods, and other found objects.

Toolbox for Recovery

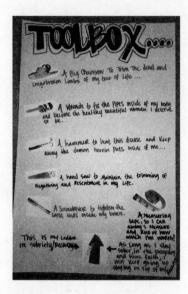

Location: Indoors

Time: 60–90 minutes

Materials: Drawing paper

Pens, pencils, or markers

Scissors

Glue or glue sticks

Pictures of actual tools
or Toolbox for Recovery
Handout

Objectives

- To have clients think creatively about what coping tools they will need to stay sober.

- To have fun with the idea of a recovery toolbox and consider which real tools they could use symbolically.

Directions

1. Before the session, prepare enough copies or photos of tools for everyone to use. The Toolbox for Recovery Handout may be copied, or tool catalogs and do-it-yourself magazines can be used. Also images of tools can be found online.

2. Introduce the concept of the recovery toolbox, which means having an assortment of good coping skills to use in stressful situations. These tools might be used to avoid triggers, manage cravings, deal with depression and frustration, or leave a risky situation. Add that having a recovery toolbox is a common term in treatment.

3. Propose the idea that an actual toolbox or tool chest is filled with real tools (hammers, nails, saws, wrenches, flashlights, measuring tapes, levels, drills—be creative here). Ask participants, "How could a hammer be used in recovery? How could a ladder be used?"

4. Ask participants to cut a collection of tools from the pictures available, or draw their own, and glue them on a piece of paper.

5. Direct participants to write how each tool could be used to help them in their recovery.

6. At the end, invite volunteers to present their ideas.

Observations

This activity was originally developed to appeal to male participants. When the idea was presented to women, they were immediately interested and joined in. Some created posters and one woman formed an actual box from paper and filled it with her tools. The participants had no difficulty grasping the concept that tools are metaphors for behavioral changes and expressed inspiring interpretations of challenges they may meet along the way.

Inspired by: A trip to the hardware store.

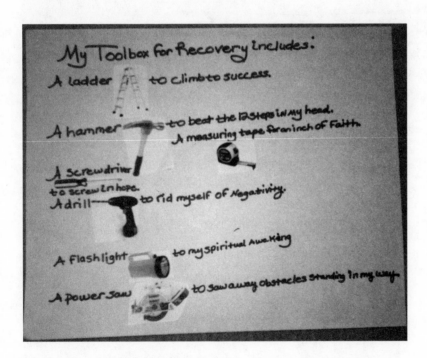

"My Toolbox for Recovery Includes:

A ladder to climb to success. A hammer to beat the 12 Steps in my head. A measuring tape for an inch of Faith. A screwdriver to screw in hope. A drill to rid myself of negativity. A flashlight to my spiritual awakening. A power saw to saw away obstacles in my way."

Toolbox for Recovery HANDOUT

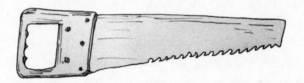

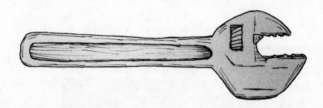

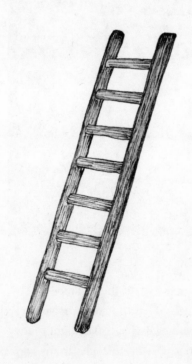

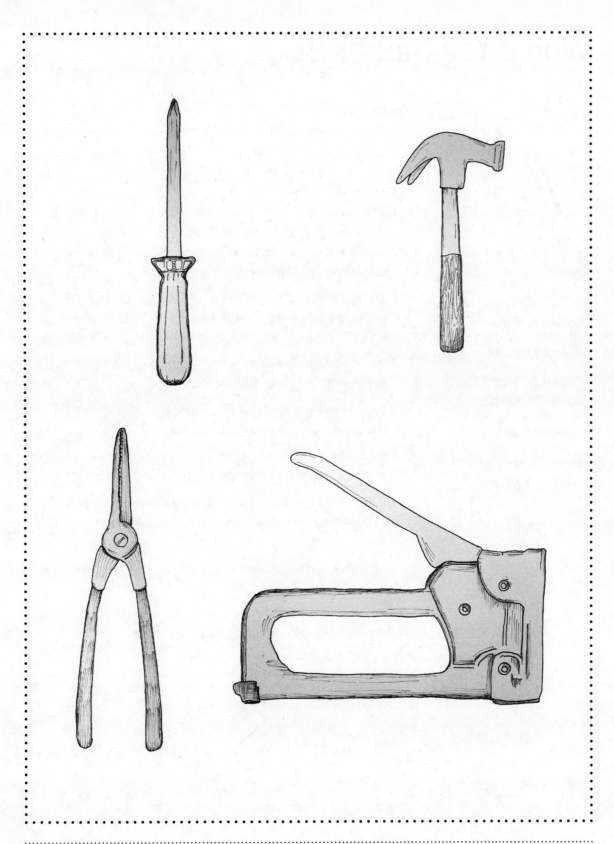

Would You Rather Be

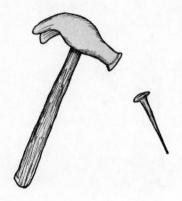

Location: Indoors

Time: 60 minutes

Materials: Would You Rather Be Handout

Drawing paper

Pens, markers, colored pencils, or crayons

Objectives

- To use metaphorical images to better understand values and qualities about the self.

Directions

1. Explain to participants that the purpose of the activity is to discover things about oneself. There are no right or wrong answers. By exploring different perspectives we all learn, especially about ourselves.

2. Using the Would You Rather Be Handout, pose the first question to the group: "Would you rather be a hammer or a nail?"

3. Allow one member of the group who prefers "hammer" to explain why he or she has that preference.

4. Ask the group if anyone prefers to be a "nail," and ask the participant to explain his or her reasons.

5. Continue to ask the rest of the questions, and permit volunteers from the group to explain their preferences.

6. After all the questions have been read aloud, invite participants to pose their own dichotomous questions to the group.

7. After the discussion, have participants think about a metaphor that is meaningful to their recovery and then draw a picture of it.

8. After allowing time for the artwork, invite participants to share their art and talk about the image they chose.

Observations

This activity was done in two groups, one that had ten people and one that had twenty-five. The larger group seemed to generate more creative ideas. The question about the tree root and branch raised deep philosophical questions. After answering four or five questions prepared by the facilitator, the group created their own. The list on the handout includes some of the ideas that prompted dynamic discussion. The participants came up with their own dichotomous ideas and made creative artwork supporting their imagery. One gave an elaborate explanation of why she preferred circle over square. One person made a three-dimensional sofa and explained that the sofa frame supported the whole of her. Another showed a nail as a linchpin that held her recovery together. Overall, this activity was fast paced and much enjoyed.

Inspired by: Simon & Garfunkle's *El Condor Pasa (If I Could)*, 1970 Sony Music Entertainment Inc.

Would You Rather Be HANDOUT

Metaphor Questions

Would you rather be a hammer or a nail?

Would you rather be a mountain or a valley?

Would you rather be a nickel or a dime?

Would you rather be a sandal or a shoe?

Would you rather be a pillow or a blanket?

Would you rather be the sun or the moon?

Would you rather be the rain or the sunshine?

Would you rather be a train or a car?

Would you rather be a pencil or an eraser?

Would you rather be a song or a guitar?

Would you rather be a tree branch or a tree root?

Would you rather be a butterfly or a bee?

Would you rather be a circle or a square?

"Normal, novel, creative, and stressful psychosocial activities in everyday life turn on patterns of activity-dependent gene expression and brain plasticity."

ERNEST ROSSI

Self-Responsibility: Emotional Regulation of Self Care

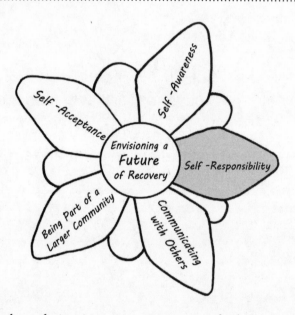

Emotional regulation is an important part of relapse prevention. Triggers and cravings may cause a person to become overwhelmed and subsequently use alcohol and other drugs again. In a similar way, emotions can easily overwhelm a person in early recovery and precipitate a return to old patterns of coping or avoidance. In this section, the activities "Erasing Triggers," "Fear in a Basket," "Serenity Boxes," and "In a Jam" teach how to face uncomfortable feelings, practice grounding skills, and develop more appropriate coping responses.

Several of the activities, such as the "Breathing Exercises," "Mindfulness Moment," "Mindful Yoga," "Sensory Meditations," "Sensory Tangerine," and "Journaling in Recovery" increase awareness in the moment and the ability to tune into feelings, sensations, and cognitions. With this increased awareness, rational decision making can be employed to challenge automatic thoughts and to consider possible responses to cues or triggers. The next logical step is taking responsibility for one's subsequent actions and behaviors.

Kay: Personally, I have used various meditation techniques successfully throughout the years for stress reduction. I am passionate about helping others, especially those with no background in meditative practice, discover ways to manage anxiety and racing thoughts. I continually find mindfulness-based activities a useful addition to my work with clients facing addictions, anxiety, trauma, and depression. The activities presented in this section are easy to understand and can be used virtually any time for quick and effective stress management, relapse prevention, and overall wellness.

One of the first times I met Roxanna, she did "Sensory Tangerine" with my caseload group. My clients were completely engaged, and one said she would never look at a tangerine in the same way again. I saw firsthand how my clients benefited from slowing down their thinking, improving their focus, and deepening their awareness, all from the ordinary action of eating a citrus fruit.

Roxanna: The activities in this section offer techniques to foster increasing capacities for distress tolerance and building healthy expectations for the future. Clients can learn to use simple methods to endure uncomfortable emotions or troublesome conditions without escaping into self-destructive behaviors. Self-awareness is increased, and the focus goes in a more positive direction.

An example of this is the "Sensory Tangerine" activity, which was done in a busy cafeteria. Instead of the noise interfering with focus, it had the effect of deepening concentration. The simultaneous actions of attending to one's own needs, remembering past experiences, and deferred gratification elevated the meaning of the experience.

Breathing Exercises

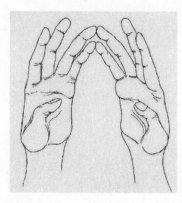

Objectives

- To teach mindful meditative breathwork for stress management through a simple exercise.

- To enhance connectedness with one's own physical body.

- To help manage anxiety.

Directions

1. Have a brief discussion about stress management and relaxation techniques, explaining that breathwork is an easy, available way to calm oneself. Read aloud the following explanation:

   The first thing we do when we are born is take a breath; the last thing we do at the end of our life is take a breath. We are all able to breathe, and it is a useful method for grounding, slowing down, or reconnecting with ourselves in the present moment. When we are stressed or panicked, our breathing is shallow and fast. To take slow, deep breaths from the belly will trigger our natural relaxation response.

2. Present more than one option for participants to try, as they may feel more comfortable with one technique.

3. Give permission to have eyes open or closed, to stay sitting on chairs, or to sit on the floor or lie down (if feasible). Unless specified, breathe through either nose or mouth.

4. Demonstrate five techniques for learning to regulate breathing. The techniques appear at the end of the directions.

5. Encourage participants to find one technique that is the easiest and the best fit for them. Encourage practicing it up to three or four times a day, or whenever they detect stress or anxiety.

Location: Indoors or Outdoors

Time: 10–30 minutes

Materials: None

Breathing Techniques

1. Diaphragmatic Breathing

- *Stand tall or sit tall with one or both hands on your belly.*

- *Take a deep, slow breath in. See and feel your belly rise as you inhale.*

- *Hold for a moment.*

- *Exhale slowly, watching and feeling your hand(s) move down in response to your belly deflating.*

- *Repeat four or five times.*

2. Four Square Window

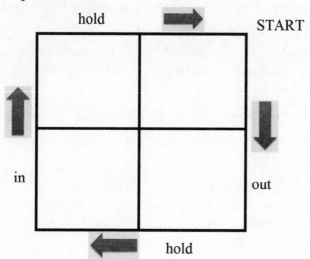

- *Imagine a square suspended in space in front of you like an imaginary window.*

- *Let your eyes trace the shape of the window, the four sides, going clockwise.*

- *Start at the upper right corner, and as you breath out, move your eyes down the right-hand border of the window, going from top to bottom, and count as you exhale, 1-2-3-4.*

- *Hold your breath, 1-2-3-4, as your eyes look along the bottom frame of the window, moving toward the next corner, hold your breath, 1-2-3-4.*

- *When you reach the third corner, breathe in, 1-2-3-4, as your eyes move along the left side going up.*

- *Now you are on the top left-hand corner, hold your breath, 1-2-3-4, as your eyes trace along the top from left to right, exhaling when you reach the corner.*

- *When you reach the upper-right-hand corner, repeat the process.*

- *At the end of the second round, rest, yawn, and notice the refreshing feeling of oxygen circulating within your body.*

3. Five Count Finger Technique

- *Hold your hands in front of you, all fingers touching but the palms apart.*

- *Breathe out, 1-2-3-4-5, and with each number, open the touch of one finger. On the count of 1 open your thumbs, and on 5, open your pinkies.*

- *Next, breath in on the count of 1-2-3-4-5, with each number reconnect the fingers, first the pinkies, up to your thumbs.*

- *Now hold the breath, 1-2-3-4-5. With each count of a number, tap the corresponding fingers together.*

- *Repeat the breathing out and the rest of the sequence.*

- *After two rounds, rest and notice the way your focus of attention has changed.*

4. Count Breaths

- *Breathe in to a count of 5 (or whatever number is comfortable for slow, deep breathing).*

- *Then breathe out longer, to a count of 7 (or whatever is comfortable). Focus on the breath going in and out.*

- *Repeat 10 times.*

5. Three-Second Relaxer

- *Take a deep breath in through your nose. Hold it for 3 seconds, 1-2-3.*

- *Then, as you let your breath out through your mouth, all at once, let your jaw and shoulders relax. Hang loose and continue breathing easily.*

- *Repeat two more times.*

Observations

In one of our groups of thirty-seven participants, about 30 percent tried all five methods. We gave them permission to participate only when and if they felt it would be of benefit. Many participants were not familiar with breathwork and were pleased to have another coping skill. It was helpful to tell participants they should choose a method that works for them and that there is not a single right way. Closing one's eyes is always optional as some trauma victims find this unsettling. Many participants reported feeling markedly relaxed after the session. The visual "Four Square Window" seemed to work with those who could envision it in their imagination. "Five Fingers" worked well for those with more of a tactile orientation. Both of those seemed to require more focus than the "Diaphragmatic Breathing" technique, but the focus of attention seemed to enhance the described benefits. There was a fairly even split for preferences of one method over another. Breathwork can be used in combination with another short activity or with a series of short activities.

Inspired by: Various relaxation, meditation, and pranayama techniques we have done personally.

Erasing Triggers

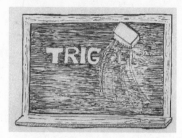

Location: Indoors

Time: 30–45 minutes

Materials: Whiteboard

Dry-erase markers

Objectives

- To help participants examine triggers associated with relapsing on alcohol and other drugs.

- To practice creative problem solving as a coping skill.

- To symbolically erase one's triggers.

Directions

1. Gather group in an auditorium or space that has a whiteboard and dry-erase markers.

2. Ask for a volunteer to come up and write on the board: first name and a personal trigger for relapse.

3. Ask other group members to offer suggestions of how this person might handle this trigger.

4. Ask the volunteer to list all suggestions on the board. Or the facilitator can do the writing.

5. Direct the volunteer to consider all the suggestions and to circle the most useful ones.

6. Allow for an interval of discussion as to how the suggestions might be helpful.

7. Tell the volunteer to take the eraser and wipe out their trigger.

8. Clean the board in preparation for next volunteer.

9. Invite another volunteer to come up to the board.

10. Continue until each participant has had an opportunity to experience the group suggestions and support.

Observations

This activity was good practice for people to walk through their triggers and consider alternatives for healthy responses. Suggestions ranged from realistic to fanciful. Overall, it was a good rehearsal of future projection for confronting risk factors outside the treatment center. At times, when common triggers were identified, it was challenging for the larger group to maintain focus on the volunteer at the board as so many wanted to actively participate in the discussion. We suggest having two facilitators in larger groups so individual attention can be offered as needed.

Inspired by: Activity designed in a different context that was described by psychotherapist Stephen Lankton, MSW, LCSW.

Exercise Circle

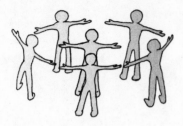

Location: Outdoors

Time: 30 minutes

Materials: Strips of paper prepared from Exercise Circle Handout

Chairs for disabled clients

Objectives

- To provide physical activity.
- To give an opportunity for cooperative leadership.
- To enhance teamwork.

Directions

1. Before the session, locate an outdoor space where there is room for the group to spread out in a circle. Also copy the Exercise Circle Handout and cut into strips of paper.

2. Instruct participants to form a circle facing inward, allowing enough space between each other so each person can reach out to the sides without hitting the next person.

3. Ask participants to choose three slips of paper with an exercise assignment. In larger groups, one slip may be sufficient.

4. Have each participant read his or her own exercises silently and, if necessary, ask for help understanding how to do the exercise.

5. Instruct one person to step into the center of the circle to demonstrate the exercise and then lead the whole group in that exercise. The leader chooses the number of repetitions. Example: Kick forward. The leader demonstrates and then announces, "We will do ten kicks with the right leg and then ten kicks with the left leg." The leader must do all the requested repetitions along with the group.

6. Direct the participant adjacent to the leader to step forward and lead one of his or her exercises, again choosing the desired number of repetitions. Leadership proceeds around the circle in a clockwise manner until each person has led an exercise.

7. Continue with a second round. Each participant will use another one of his or her three slips.

8. On the third round, instruct the leader to use the exercise on the final strip, or to choose his or her favorite exercise. The leader can call out any exercise to do regardless of whether it has been done before. Example: "Deep knee bends. Do twenty-five!"

Observations

"Exercise Circle" was performed several times on sunny days with a group of thirty. This activity offers a way to appropriately exhibit talents, channel aggressive tendencies, or express disappointment or discontent in a friendly, supportive atmosphere. The activity gives visual demonstrations of adapting exercises to meet personal needs and role modeling of participatory behavior by non-athletic staff members. Empirical evidence suggests dance movement therapies can be an integral part of a healing process, and we wanted to have an activity that incorporated expressive movement. The combination of physical activity in a structured format invited positive participation and gave an opportunity for those who are not as outspoken to take leadership and to make choices that affect the group as a whole. The experience brought out cooperative support and enhanced group cohesiveness. The activity provided a forum for some of the self-isolating participants to demonstrate their skills in a positive way. We had an interest in increasing the physical activity of the residents, who were often very sedentary. Since the average athletic ability of the group was poor, participation by an older member of the professional staff illustrated the achievability of the tasks requested. The final round, in which creative or preferred exercises were chosen, showed a diverse response ranging from very easy (Deep breaths, take three) to challenging (Lunges, do 20 with each leg). Participation was inclusive and good-natured, with some calling out "Oh no!" but proceeding with the exercise. The group had to be reminded not to have personal conversations during exercises, and leaders had to speak loudly to be heard.

Inspired by: Recollections of elementary school physical education. We were encouraged by the idea of movement behavior in the therapeutic relationship and the healing through movement advocated by the American Dance Therapy Association and other similar groups.

Exercise Circle HANDOUT

Cut the following into individual slips.

Whirlwind one arm in-front, up and around, right, then left, then both

Whirlwind both arms by your side, up and around,
clockwise then counter-clockwise

Kick front, right leg, then left leg

Kick side, right leg, then left leg

Ankle twist, right then left

Waist bend, hands on hips

Waist circles, clockwise, then counter-clockwise

Move from waist, arms stretched out, turn shoulders to right, then left

Pat you own back over your head, right then left

Pat your own back reaching upward from waist, right then left

Turn face, side to side

Look up, look down

Lunge, front knee bent, back knee straight, right then left

Kick own butt, right leg, then left leg

Hip circles, clockwise then counter-clockwise

Make yourself tall

Clap hands behind you, at waist, then overhead

Elbows up, chicken flap forward and back

Hold your foot up to waist in front, right then left

Hold foot up to butt with opposite hand, right then left

Hold hands overhead, bend at waist front and back

Hold hands overhead and bend at waist, side to side

Hold breath to count of five, then breathe out slow

Waist bend hands behind you, front then back

Punch from waist right hand, then left, then both

Imaginary rowing motion

Stand on tiptoes, hands at sides, stretch your spine

Two-feet bunny hop, then one-foot hop

March in place, knees high

Lift imaginary heavy barbell, up from floor over your head

Flex your bicep with one hand on hip, and other in the air, right then left

Put on imaginary shorts, one leg and then the other, pull them up

Put on imaginary t-shirt over your head, put on one arm and then the other arm

Knee to chest, right then left

Touch toes, feet together, knees straight

Hands touch the ground, legs wide

Sideways motion, one leg bent, one straight, head and back upright

Shrug shoulders round about, front then back

Knee bends

Reach for the sky

Touch elbows behind you

Jumping jacks

Jump forward, jump back

Pull tummy way in

Stretch and yawn

"Teach them to be comfortable in their bodies."

MILTON H. ERICKSON

Fear in a Basket

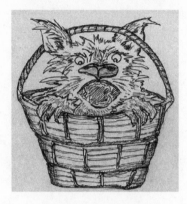

Location: Indoors or Outdoors

Time: 30–45 minutes (based on number of people)

Materials: Index cards

Pens

Basket

Objectives

- To provide a safe, nonjudgmental arena to discuss fears and insecurities about maintaining recovery.

Directions

1. Distribute one index card and a pen to each participant.

2. Instruct participants to *anonymously* write their greatest fear or worry about actually being sober. (Something other than relapsing.)

3. Encourage participants to be as specific and as honest as possible.

4. After everyone is done writing a fear or worry, ask them to fold the card in half and deposit in a small basket.

5. Mix up the cards.

6. Pass the basket around so each participant takes one card. The card must be from another participant.

7. Ask participants to take turns reading aloud each fear. Each reader attempts to explain what the person who wrote it might mean.

8. After all fears have been read and elaborated, discuss fears common to the whole group.

Observations

This activity was done successfully many times with small process groups of approximately six to twelve. It helped to build trust and unity, as people came to realize that most everyone has similar fears. This activity could lead to a discussion of a team or caseload contract, or goals the group wishes to achieve.

Inspired by: A common icebreaker activity in workshops.

"The pain is the push,
the vision is the pull."

PATRICK CARNES

Find Your Identity Groups

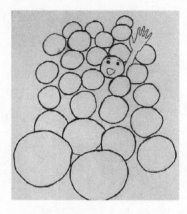

Location: Indoors or Outdoors

Time: 25 minutes

Materials: Find Your Identity Groups Handout

Objectives

- To familiarize participants with the concept of identity groups and with the multitude of ways that communication is expressed nonverbally.

- To provide a venue for individuals to recognize they are not alone.

Directions

1. Begin with a brief discussion of purpose. Read aloud the following explanation:

   Each person belongs to a number of groups. Among these groups are race, education, religion, age, and other factors that define who we are. Some we may have worked for and are proud of, like having job skills, education, or children; others we have less control over, including race, age, or even family status. Our identity is a unique and personal constellation of different features. Our awareness of the various groups to which we belong often provides an automatic opportunity to bond with others or is, conversely, a barrier to the ways that we communicate. Becoming aware of our own identity, and the degree to which we embrace and accept certain factors about ourselves, can help us to connect with some people and help us to distance ourselves from others. The process involves not only self-awareness but also awareness of the subtle ways in which information and values are communicated.

2. Explain to participants that they will listen to questions and communicate nonverbally, moving around the group together with others who answer the question the same way. They are finding their own identity group. Emphasize there is no correct answer to any question.

3. Demonstrate with four volunteers. Only body language can be used—no talking, no nodding, no thumbs up, or other gestures allowed. Eye contact is permitted.

4. Say aloud, *"Do you think you will be successful in recovery?"* "Yes" group and "No" group find each other and gather in two clusters.

5. On completion of the demonstration, begin the activity by reading aloud a question from the list. Participants are expected to gather into two clusters depending on each person's answer to the question. The questions are dichotomous, meaning that the answers fall into two categories.

6. Once the groups have formed after each question, say, *"Raise your hand if your answer is _____"* so participants can see whether or not they have joined with the correct group of peers.

7. Continue to read aloud the questions on the list.

8. When the larger group is successful in finding peers, make the activity more complex by using the questions that have multiple potential answers.

Observations

This activity was done in a community college setting with eighteen freshman, and with groups of more than thirty in a recovery setting. In all cases, the majority of the participants became engaged, while several sat on the periphery not involved. As different questions were posed, more individuals participated until nearly full participation was achieved. It was a fairly rapid interval before the dichotomous questions were too easy due to increasing awareness of nonverbal signals. This activity made a good warm-up for a discussion about identification of substance-abuse triggers.

Inspired by: Game at a child's birthday party.

Find Your Identity Groups HANDOUT

(Questions 1–15 have two possible answers.)

1. Is this your first time in recovery? *Yes / No*

2. Did you go into recovery on your own, or were you forced by legal issues or loved ones? *Own / Others*

3. Do you know where you will live after leaving this treatment center? *Have a home / Still looking*

4. Do you have a sponsor? *Still looking / Have sponsor*

5. Do you think you will have the same sponsor next year that you will have when you leave treatment? *Same sponsor / Different one*

6. Do you plan for ninety meetings in ninety days? *Plan on it / Undecided*

7. Did you have a home group before you got to treatment? *Had home group / Didn't have*

8. Have you started on the Twelve Steps before? *First time / Started before*

9. Have you ever you had a successful twelve months of sobriety? *Never had a year / Had before*

10. Do you remember what clean and sober really feels like? *Don't remember / Do remember*

11. Do you expect you will struggle with triggers and cravings next month? *Yes / No*

12. Do you know what sort of a job you want to have this time next year? *Still figuring / Yes*

13. Do you have friends who are supportive of your recovery? *Yes / No*

14. Have you sat outside in the sunshine in the last two days? *Yes / No*

15. Have you ever been homeless? *Yes / No*

(Questions 16–25 have multiple possible answers.)

16. What type of twelve-step group will you join? *AA / NA / Both / Something else*

17. How many times have you been in recovery? *1 / 2 / 3 / 4 / More*

18. When you get out of inpatient treatment where will you live? *Where I lived before / Transitional housing / Don't know / Homeless*

19. How long is the longest you have been in recovery ? *Never before now / Three months / Six months / One year / More than two years*

20. How connected are you with your home group? *Feel certain it's the right group for me / Hopeful it will work out but uncertain / Don't really want to go to meetings*

21. What kind of job do you hope to get? *Something I've worked in before / Need new training / No ideas*

22. How do you feel about your progress in recovery? *The worst is over / I worry things will get worse / No idea*

23. What is your progress in working the Twelve Steps? *Haven't started / Completed Step One / Completed Step Two or Step Three*

24. What kind of people were you hanging out with before you arrived here? *Users / Sober people / I kept to myself*

25. Do you have a clear vision of your sober self in the future? *One day at a time / One month / One year / Ten years*

In a Jam

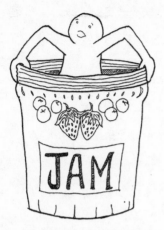

Location: Indoors or Outdoors

Time: 60 minutes

Materials: In a Jam Handout (cut into small pieces of paper)

Jar, basket, or bag

Objectives

- To demonstrate problem solving techniques for common, everyday problems.

- To elicit group feedback regarding the appropriateness and the effectiveness of each strategy.

- To encourage cooperation and group work.

Directions

1. Before the session, make a copy of the In a Jam Handout and cut into strips. Place strips in a jar, a small basket, or a bag so participants can choose one at a time.

2. Review instructions with group and demonstrate as needed.

3. Allow participants to work individually or as teams of two or more. Each participant or team draws a scenario from the container. Give each participant or group a few minutes to think or discuss. Then each participant or group takes turns coming up to the front.

4. Ask the participant or group to read aloud the scenario.

5. Direct the participant or group to demonstrate both the unhealthy and the healthy way of responding to the situation, commenting on which response might have used in the past.

6. Invite the whole group to give feedback on the effectiveness of handling the situation.

7. Ask the next participant or group to repeat the activity, choosing a new scenario.

8. Continue as time allows.

Observations

This was a successful activity in many groups, both large and small. It was used several times as part of an anger management process group and elicited active dialogue filled with humor and practical advice. Participants embraced the opportunity to express their honest reactions and to contrast their own impulsive responses with ones that were more appropriate. The audience response supported active and adaptive learning. In a larger group, the activity was enjoyed and brought forth creative problem solving for situations common to the group-living experience. On another occasion, this activity was adapted for a Seeking Safety group and renamed "In a Pickle," in which various scenarios related to safety were constructed and responded to.

Inspired by: Childhood games.

In A Jam Scenarios HANDOUT

Cut out and put in jar, bag, or basket.

Your roommate bounces a ball in the house even after you ask him to stop.

You are always the one stuck doing the dishes.

Someone cuts in front of you in line at a store.

You bang your toe on something in a public place with others around you.

The clerk at the grocery store is rude for no reason.

You order food at a restaurant but don't like it.

You have been waiting for a really long time to be served in a restaurant.

A friend asks if you like the shirt she is wearing, but you hate the color.

It's time to leave, but you can't find your keys. Your significant other pitches in to help but says that you are always losing things.

You're walking along a crowded walkway and bump shoulders with a stranger going in the other direction.

Your neighbor is playing music for hours, and it's really loud.

You do a week's grocery shopping and when in line you realize your wallet is at home.

One neighbor on your block doesn't mow the lawn. The grass is really high.

Someone asks to borrow cigarette money, and you know you won't be paid back.

Someone takes your last cigarette.

Someone unjustly accuses you of borrowing a pair of jeans.

Someone borrows your favorite
pen and does not return it.

Someone shoplifts, and
you let it happen.

You get disconnected in the middle
of a really important call.

You are on the phone to a company
and spend a long time on hold.

Someone says something
insulting to you.

Everyone is laughing, and
you don't get the joke.

You are asked to read aloud in
group but don't feel like it.

Class runs late, and you are tired of it.

Someone you don't know
keeps looking at you.

You want to smoke, but you
are in a no smoking area.

You let your friend borrow your car, and
it is returned with an empty gas tank.

You're on the bus and a smelly
person sits next to you.

You're finished chewing your gum
and don't see a waste basket.

Someone is whispering, and you think
the person is talking about you.

Your have a doctor visit, and
the doctor rushes you and does
not treat you with respect.

You break a vase that belongs to
someone else, but no one saw you do it.

Someone is trying to explain something,
but you know more about the topic.

You loaned a book to someone,
but it was never returned,
and you want it now.

At dinner, a friend makes a big
deal about not being able to
eat anything on the menu.

The group wants to sit outside
in the sunshine, but you prefer
the air conditioning.

Your neighbor's dog won't stop barking.

The group leader calls on the same person in the group over and over.

At dinner, a friend reaches over and takes a bite off your plate without asking.

A friend is talking too much, and you have something you need to work on and concentrate.

You have a very important phone call, and someone is ahead of you tying up the phone.

You go to a wedding reception, and people keep offering you a glass of champagne.

A lady with a crying baby sits on the other end of the park bench where you went for peace and quiet.

You're at the movies, and someone behind you is talking in loud whispers.

You set aside a special piece of cake in the refrigerator, and your roommate eats it.

An old boyfriend or girlfriend keeps calling, and you don't want to talk.

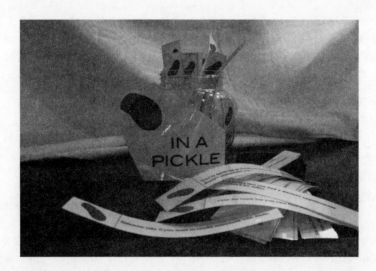

The "In a Pickle" variation on this activity.

"Not knowing the outcome is one of the critical risks of courage."

Patrick Carnes

Journaling in Recovery

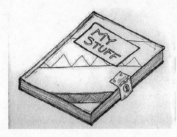

Location: Indoors

Time: 60–90 minutes

Materials: 8 ½" × 11" cardstock in various colors

Pieces of 8 ½" × 11" colored paper (cut in half)

Hole puncher

Yarn, string, ribbon, or brad fasteners

Markers

Decorative materials

Journaling in Recovery Handout (one per person)

Objectives

- To introduce or reinforce journaling as an adaptive coping strategy.

- To provide an environment to create a personalized journal even if there are limited resources.

Directions

1. Discuss the merits and purposes of keeping a journal, referring to the Journaling in Recovery Handout.

2. Encourage participants who have journaled in the past to discuss their process.

3. Have participants choose a cardstock cover for their journal and approximately ten sheets of colored paper.

4. Instruct participants to punch holes in the side of paper and insert between the front and back covers.

5. Tell participants to fasten the pages and covers with yarn, string, or brad fasteners.

6. After the construction of the journal is complete, tell participants the journal can be organized or decorated as desired.

7. Encourage participants to write their first entry.

8. Ask volunteers to share their finished journals.

Observations

While some participants already kept journals, everyone enjoyed this activity. Some created books to keep medication logs, and some made gratitude or Step Ten books. Whether participants actually envisioned themselves using the book did not seem to impact the enjoyment.

Inspired by: Keeping journals through the years and making books as a child.

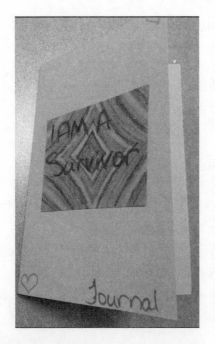
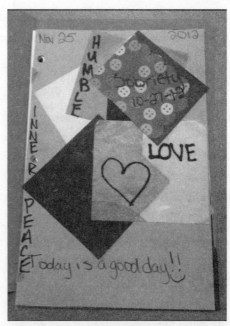
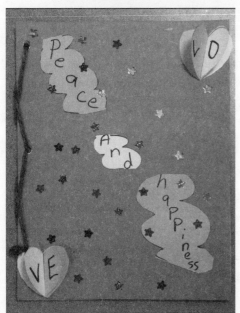
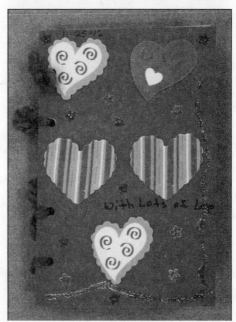

An assortment of journals created in the group, all with positive messages to self.

Journaling in Recovery HANDOUT

Keep a journal or diary to have a record of moments of gratitude, goals, intentions, and the ups and the downs of life. Use it as a daily personal inventory. Sometimes writing about what is bothersome in our journal makes us feel better. When we can go back and read our concerns or goals, we can make clear, focused choices of what works for us and what has not.

Journaling is all about self-expression. Recording our feelings, recognizing them, and leaving them on the page is an excellent way to understand and figure out what is really important to us and for us. We realize what we are really experiencing. We see what we are really thinking. It is right there on the page in black and white. Where is the fear? Where is the joy? Keeping an addiction recovery journal can reduce stress and help us focus and organize. It can be a good reminder of things to accomplish and can be useful to set and track goals.

Journaling Tips

1. Start journaling on any day of the year.

2. Put your journal where you see it every day, such as next to your bed, on the kitchen table, or on your desk. This will help remind you to journal daily.

3. Keep a pen or pencil with your journal.

4. Skipping days is a part of journaling. It's okay.

5. You can use the same color of pen or use different colors. You can also use certain colors of pens for certain feelings, e.g., green for growth, blue for sadness, orange for joy, or red for anger. If you are using different colored pens, write in the front of your journal what each color means.

6. Start by writing about anything. If you need help getting started, try answering any or all of these questions:

   - How am I feeling? How do I want to be feeling? What do I want to learn about myself?

   - What do I want to change? What would I never change about myself?

   - What are some of my goals?

   - Describe the room.

   - Describe the people in your life.

   - Describe yourself.

- Describe something beautiful you can see or hear.

- Describe how you would like things to be one month from now and one year from now.

Digital Journals

If you have access to a smartphone or computer, there are many apps (many are free, some are just a couple of dollars) that allow you to journal anytime. If you are out and you have a thought you want to journal about right away, or you find writing with pen and paper frustrating, this may work well for you. Some of the apps allow you to dictate your thoughts to make the writing easier. Other apps allow you to choose paper, fonts, colors, and add photos so it can look like a real journal.

Milk Art

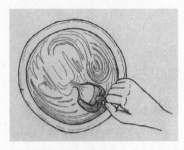

Location: Indoors

Time: 15–20 minutes

Materials: Small container of milk

Saucer (one per person)

Cotton swabs

Food coloring

Dish detergent

Several small bowls

Paper plates

Water

Objectives

- To note fleeting changes and unexpected ways in which factors influence the direction of energy.

- To provide a backdrop for further discussion of how outside influences affect addiction and recovery.

Directions

1. Pass out saucers, paper plates, and cotton swabs.

2. Place small bowls with about a quarter cup of water and a few drops of detergent where several people can use them.

3. Have participants use paper plates to hold saucers and used cotton swabs.

4. Pass out milk, just enough in each saucer to create a smooth surface.

5. Instruct participants to sprinkle drops of food coloring in the milk.

6. Direct participants to dip the cotton swabs in the detergent mix and then touch the surface of the milk.

7. Discuss what kind of amazing varied and beautiful designs emerge.

Observations

The context of creating a transient, but beautiful, work of art was used as a springboard for discussion. After participants enjoyed exploring the effects, the facilitator transitioned into the ways that unanticipated factors can impact the design of one's life.

Inspired by: Dr. Rubin Battino, Professor Emeritus of Chemistry at Wright State University and licensed counselor.

"To become whole, to be in harmony, to be centered, to find one's true self, to be at peace with yourself, and the world—all of these are manifestations of healing."

RUBIN BATTINO

Mindfulness Moment

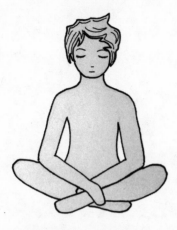

Location: Indoors

Time: 30–45 minutes

Materials: None

Objectives

- To introduce the concept of mindfulness, which is paying close attention to your present moment in a nonjudgemental way.

- To encourage self-awareness of any physical sensations, emotions, and automatic thoughts that may be present in the moment.

Directions

1. Discuss meditation and how it can be something other than clearing the mind or thinking about nothing. Read aloud the following explanation:

   There are always thoughts, emotions, and sensations in our bodies and our minds. Paying close attention to what is happening to us in the current moment can promote greater awareness. This greater awareness can be a coping skill to help with relapse prevention. We can learn to catch ourselves at the beginning of a craving or urge or when we start to feel overwhelmed if we are more tuned in to what we are feeling and thinking.

2. Invite participants to sit comfortably on the floor or chair. Read aloud the following guided meditation:

   Take a moment to adjust your position comfortably sitting in the chair or on the floor, if that's more comfortable. Gently closing your eyes if you wish and settling into your body . . . . If it's more comfortable for you not to close your eyes, just keep a soft focus a few feet in front of you. If you are sitting, ensure your body is upright and comfortable for you, or if you are lying down, feel comfortable and safe. Now, in your own way, take a few moments to relax your body . . . . Taking a deliberate, deep breath. Perhaps feeling the muscles softening and loosening . . . If there are any areas of tightness and tension, just notice that and try to breath into that area. Now taking another deep breath, slowly breathe in and out.

Just relaxing and releasing. Simply letting go. As you breathe out, notice that natural feeling of relaxing and releasing a little more with each out breath. Just simply letting go.

If your mind wanders to other thoughts, this is okay, this is what minds do. Just notice that and gently bring your attention to your breath. In through nose, filling your lungs and filling your belly. Perhaps notice a gently rising of the belly. Then releasing the breath, the belly flattens and the breath flows out.

Now pay attention to any sounds outside the room. Just listening . . . with a gentle curiosity . . . letting the sounds come and go . . . no need to judge . . . just noticing.

Now notice any sounds that may be coming from inside the room. Notice the sound of your own breathing . . . even if very soft . . . just listening . . . just noticing.

Bringing your awareness to your breath, notice what sensations are there as you breathe in . . . and as you breathe out . . . feeling the air touch your nostrils . . . feeling the slight movement of your chest and belly . . . listening to the gentle sound of your own breathing . . . allowing your breath to take up whatever rhythm feels natural for you at the moment. No need to force it, just breathe easily. If you notice your attention wandering or becoming distracted, simply bring your attention back to the next inbreath.

Be aware of the next breath . . . and the next breath. Be aware of what it is breathing in . . . and breathing out. Simply being with the breath . . . aware of the breath.

Now very slowly and gently, still maintaining an awareness of your body, when you are ready, move the body a little, wiggling the fingers and toes or gently stretching. Allow your eyes to open and your awareness to include the room and the people around you.

3. Allow for an interval of becoming reacclamated to the surroundings.

4. Elicit feedback by asking questions, such as, "How was that for you?" and "What did you notice? Any thoughts? Any emotions? Any physical sensations?" Avoid judging any comment as good or bad.

Observations

Most clients found this activity relaxing. Some who were agitated or hyperaroused had difficulty sitting still, but they were reassured this was fine and was something to notice about themselves that day. Some clients fell asleep, but they were told they still would receive the benefits of the relaxation. It is best, however, for participants to stay awake, and even stand to increase wakefulness.

Inspired by: Workshops in Mindfulness-Based Stress Reduction, Mindfulness-Based Relapse Prevention, and Mindfulness-Based Cognitive Therapy.

"Mindful awareness of our emotions, thoughts, and physical sensations helps us manage moments of suffering and have more pleasure in the pleasant moments."

KAY COLBERT

Mindful Yoga

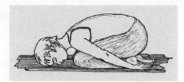

Location: Indoors or Outdoors

Time: 45 minutes

Materials: Yoga mats or bath towels (one per person)

Optional: Meditation music, prerecorded guided meditation

Objectives

- To introduce mindful meditation practice through simple movement.

- To increase awareness of the body and any physical sensations in the present moment.

Directions

1. Before the session, ask participants to wear comfortable, loose-fitting clothes and to take their shoes and socks off. If yoga mats are available, that is ideal. This class has been conducted successfully with bath towels on a grassy lawn.

2. Reassure participants that none of the poses or movements will be complicated, and the group will be conducted at a slow pace. If anyone finds a pose challenging or painful in any way, he or she should stop. Those who feel they cannot participate for whatever reason are encouraged to sit in chair and do the breathing and arm movements as best they can. Explain that this is more than exercise or stretching; it is also another coping tool for relaxation and self-awareness. Add that the only thing participants need to pay attention to is what they are doing at any given moment; this is not a competition.

3. Read aloud the following directions slowly and pause often to check that everyone understands. You may want to do only some of these positions, but be sure to start with a sitting pose and end with lying down.

   Everyone sit comfortably on your mat (towel). You may cross your legs or keep them out in front of you, whatever feels comfortable for you right now. Imagine there is a string coming out of the top of your head and reaching to the sky, gently pulling your spine straight. Feel your hips anchored into the ground. Now take a slow, deep breath from your belly and slowly let it out. Do this again, in and out, and imagine your chest and your heart opening up. Continue to breathe in and out slowly for five to ten more breaths.

Now, on the inhale, raise your arms slowly and then on the exhale, lower your arms. Let's try this again. Repeat four more times. Now come forward onto your knees, with your hands on the floor. Take a deep breath in, and on the exhale, raise your back up slowly like a cat arching its back. Then on the inhale, slowly let your back sink back down and bring your chin up. This is traditionally called the "Cat and Cow" pose. Repeat five or six times slowly.

Now let's sit down on the mat with legs out. Again imagine your head is reaching for the sky while your hips are anchored onto the ground. Breath in and imagine your spine lengthening. Turn slightly to the right and place your hands beside your right leg. Take a breath or two here, feeling just a gentle stretch. If you feel any pulling or any pain, stop. Now turn to the left, placing your hands beside your left leg and take a couple of breaths here, feeling just a gentle stretch.

Now sit up, sitting on your legs, lean forward until your hands reach the floor. Breathe in and out. This is called Child's Pose. Perhaps you can put your arms on the floor, or your head. Only go as far as is comfortable for you. Pay attention to any sensations in your body.

Now lie on your back with your knees bent. Let your knees fall to the right. Spend a moment here, just noticing what you feel in your body. Now bring your knees back to center, take a breath, and now let your knees fall to the left. Does this side feel the same or different?

Now bring your knees to your chest and hug them. Rock gently back and forth or side to side, maybe making small circles with the small of your back, giving yourself a back massage.

Now lie down on your back, legs out and relaxed. Let your arms lay beside you, palms open and turned to the ceiling. Tuck your shoulder blades under and let your head tilt back naturally. Take a deep breath in and out, letting yourself relax and be supported by the floor or the ground. Spend a few moments here, breathing gently, letting go, just being. Do a scan of your body, starting with your feet, your legs, thighs, hips, belly, chest, back, shoulders, arms, hands, neck, face, head, and top of head. What do you notice? Any areas of tightness, holding, or warmth? Just notice any sensations that come up and continue to breathe.

4. If you wish, play soothing meditation music on the last pose, or perhaps do a guided meditation or brief, guided body scan.

Observations

For some of our clients, this group was their first introduction to yoga or meditative movement. Almost all enjoyed the class and said they felt more relaxed and centered afterward. Many expressed a desire to find a regular yoga class when they left the treatment center. Be sensitive to those with trauma issues; occasionally there is a flooding of emotions, and a participant may need to take a break.

Inspired by: A variety of yoga and meditation classes taken over the years, as well as Mindfulness-Based Stress Reduction techniques.

"There can be many separate states of awareness that develop spontaneously in ordinary life."

MILTON H. ERICKSON

Trading Self-Soothing Techniques

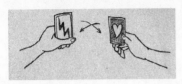

Location: Indoors

Time: 45 minutes

Materials: Blank note cards

Pens

Small basket

Self-Soothing Handout

Objectives

- To explore techniques for making oneself feel comfortable.

- To compare techniques with others.

- To increase coping strategies for adapting to stress in various ways.

Directions

1. Initiate a group discussion on the multitude of ways that individuals respond to stress. Encourage the group to consider individual techniques for dealing with stress. Responses generally fall into categories such as letting off steam, altering the situation, or otherwise soothing and comforting the stressed individual.

2. Distribute the Self-Soothing Handout and have participants select from the list of negative emotions and look at the effectiveness of their habitual responses.

3. Sequentially, ask each participant to use the sentence stem to describe his or her own coping style. For example, "When I am angry, I sometimes walk away, which usually doesn't change anything."

4. Once the participant reflects upon his or her own style of coping, pose the question, "Does this action lead you in the direction of who you want to be?"

5. Ask the next participant to use the sentence stem to reveal one of his or her own self-soothing techniques and to respond to the question, "Does this action lead you in the direction of who you want to be?"

6. Continue until all participants have spoken.

7. Upon reviewing what current strategies each participant uses, ask the participants to focus on adaptive strategies that work well for them.

8. Direct participants to take three blank note cards and write about self-soothing techniques they use to help them cope in a positive, healthy way.

9. Turn the note cards face down and pile in center of the table or place in a basket.

10. Have participants draw a card that is not theirs and read aloud the technique selected. If this is something not already used by the participant, then he or she holds on to the card.

11. Continue until each participant has at least one card identifying a technique he or she does not currently use but is willing to try.

12. Encourage participants to keep their cards and give the adaptive technique a try next time an opportunity arises.

Observations

This activity was done twice with groups of six and twelve. Several remarked they were unaware they already used such a broad repertoire. At the end of the sessions, each had a strategy in hand and expressed interest in trying something new. One who drew the strategy to "get on the computer" chose to imagine herself surfing online. The activity was well received, and all left with expressed enthusiasm.

Inspired by: Childhood games played with siblings.

Trading Self-Soothing Techniques HANDOUT

When I feel _____ (identify a stressful emotion)

I sometimes _____ (identify a coping action)
which usually (choose one) **helps, doesn't help, or makes things worse.**

Possible Stressful Emotions

Bored	Annoyed	Discontent	Worried	Upset
Bothered	Angered	Discouraged	Offended	Distrustful
Hurt	Mad	Confused	Lonely	Embarrassed
Irritated	Scared	Doubtful	Discontent	
Depressed	Frustrated	Hopeless	Grumpy	

Possible Coping Actions

Confront the other person	Hurt someone else
Run away	Hurt myself
Listen to music	Complain to others
Take a deep breath	Imagine a change
Stop, look, and listen	Exercise
Wait until later to respond	Retreat
Laugh about it	Analyze
Prove myself better	Put it in writing
Write a song about it	Go off by myself
Ignore it	Review it in my own mind
Lend a helping hand to someone else	Retaliate
Keep a list	Change the subject
Change clothes	Distract myself
Go shopping	Watch a movie
Pretend I didn't notice	Pray
Eat	Focus on what I want
Sleep	Count
Figure out the cause	Use my imagination
Feel the sunshine	Cry
Read	Picture myself somewhere else

"Life will bring you pain all by itself.
Your responsibility is to create joy."

MILTON H. ERICKSON

Sensory Meditations

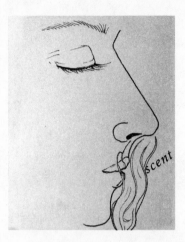

Location: Indoors or Outdoors

Time: 45–60 minutes

Materials: One of the following per person:

Collection of small rocks or pebbles in a basket or box

Cotton balls in a container

Assortment of 3 or 4 essential oils (lavender, bergamot, rosemary, lemongrass, eucalyptus, thyme)

Variety of stress balls

3 or 4 examples of meditation music/sounds (water, rain, waves, chimes, birds)

Objectives

- To educate about the benefits of meditation.

- To introduce alternative ways to meditate and find calm.

- To stimulate an array of sensory experiences for neural enrichment.

Directions

1. Before the session, collect the materials. Rocks may be found on hikes. Health food stores carry essential oils; these are used sparingly, so they last a long time. Stress balls come in a variety of shapes, sizes, and textures and may be found inexpensively at toy stores, sports stores, or online. Nature sounds can easily be downloaded and played through a speaker.

2. Proceed as you would for a group meditation. Ask everyone to sit comfortably in a chair or on the floor and settle in with a few slow, deep breaths from the belly.

3. Explain that the group will try several short (a few minutes each) meditations using different objects to focus the mind.

4. When ready to begin, read aloud the following explanation: *Each person will react differently, and there is no right or wrong way to do this. Just notice how you react to each object, and what thoughts, emotions, or physical sensations come up for you.*

Rocks: Pass around a small box or basket filled with small rocks or pebbles of various shapes and sizes. Instruct everyone to close their eyes before they take a rock and hold the rock in their closed hand without looking at it. Then ask participants to take a few slow, deep breaths and think about the rock in their hand. Ask the group: *What shape is it? Is it smooth or rough? Does it have indentations in it? What color is it? Is it all one color?* Then ask everyone to open their eyes and look at their rock. Was it what they imagined?

Essential oils: Pass around cotton balls to the group. They may take one or several. Then pass around the bottles of essential oils and instruct participants to carefully smell each one, choose one they like, and then gently put one drop on their cotton ball. Warn that essential oils are strong, one drop is enough, and it should not touch the eyes or skin as it might irritate. Alternatively, cotton balls can be pre-scented and put in small bowls or muffin tins and passed around. Ask everyone to settle in comfortably and quietly, hold the cotton ball a few inches from their nose, and breathe in the scent. Then say, *Eyes may be closed or not. Focus on the scent and whatever images or thoughts it prompts. You may like this scent or not; it may remind you of something.* You might explain that some people believe that certain scents have healing properties or can alter a person's mood, which is called aromatherapy. Suggest that participants can use this scented pad as the focus of their meditation, relaxing into the aroma.

Stress balls: Pass around an assortment of soft squeeze balls that can be held in the hand. Have enough so everyone can have one, although participants may take turns trying out the various textures and shapes. Ask everyone to take several slow, deep breaths and squeeze or roll their balls in their hands. Then say, *Think about the texture and the density. Is the ball smooth or rough? Is it thick or thin? Is the ball easy to squeeze them or is there resistance?*

Music: Explain that some people find it helpful to relax to musical sounds or nature sounds. This type of music has no words but may create pleasant pictures or stories in the mind. Encourage everyone to listen carefully to the sounds and notice what they "see" in their mind. Then play short (thirty seconds to one minute) pieces of three or four simple sounds, such as waves, rain, or crystal bowl music. Then ask for volunteers to share their experience.

Observations

This activity was done many times and worked especially well with groups of ten to twelve. Only once, a participant remarked loudly that the rock she was holding was a trigger as it reminded her of a piece of crack cocaine. This comment in turn triggered other clients, so we calmly moved on to the next part. One client, who was extremely anxious and met the criteria for DID (Dissociative Identity Disorder), found the scent meditation very calming. After learning this technique, she carried a cotton pad scented with lavender oil in her pocket and used it as a grounding tool when feeling overwhelmed. The stress balls were quite popular with clients who were agitated and would often ask to borrow the balls during the day, saying it helped them channel their feelings appropriately.

Inspired by: A client, blind from birth, who said she imagined colors as different musical tones. Also by various clients who said they had difficulty following guided meditations or sitting still. And thanks to a wonderful counselor, Deb Castillo, LPC, for the rock activity.

"Healing is accelerated when we engage multiple senses."

KAY COLBERT

Sensory Tangerine

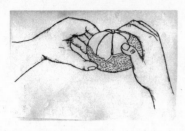

Location: Indoors or Outdoors (quiet, distraction-free environment)

Time: 20 minutes

Materials: Tangerines (select attractive, unblemished fruit; one per person)

Alternate fruit in event someone has allergy to citrus

Objectives

- To engage participants in sensory appreciation while developing patience and exercising delayed gratification.

Directions

1. Prior to passing around the tangerines, explain the purpose and the duration of the activity.

2. Explain that there will be no second helpings.

3. Ask participants to stay with the activity and not move ahead faster than instructed. Do not peel the tangerine or eat it until instructed to do so.

4. Have each participant select one tangerine for use while participating in the activity.

5. Explain that voluntary verbal feedback will be asked for at the conclusion of the activity, but there should be silence during the activity.

6. After passing out fruit, encourage holding and touching personal tangerines.

7. The sensory portion lasts about ten minutes.

8. Read aloud the script, modifying it to meet the needs of the individuals present.

9. Proceed at a slow, deliberate pace, with intentional pauses and intervals of silence.

10. Conclude with a discussion involving the feelings each person had during the process of anticipation, waiting, and enjoying. Discuss ways the passage of time seemed to move more slowly than usual.

11. Donate any leftover whole fruit to the cafeteria.

SCRIPT

Look at the tangerine.

Notice the deep rich color,

The contrast of the intense vibrant orange,

With the small jagged edge of green where the stem attaches.

The way the bumps on the skin form visible highs and lows.

Texture that can be explored even without touching it.

Are there any scars? Irregularities?

There always are.

Yet those differences do not take away from the beauty,

But rather give a picture of individuality and character.

Imagine the contrast with the white you know is on the inside of the skin,

The translucent membranes around the segments,

The yellowish white of the seeds,

The deep juicy orange color of the fruit itself.

Feel the tangerine.

Touch the skin. Notice how it is pliable, soft in its own way,

Strong enough to protect the soft, inner contents.

The flexibility, ability to bend and adjust with pressure, is part of its strength.

It has character and texture.

Maybe there are marks or imperfections.

Feel those wounds.

Appreciate the manner that the skin has healed itself and created a protective shell around the softness inside.

Smell the tangerine,

The mild fragrance of the skin.

If you have ever smelled the gentle aroma of citrus blossoms in the air,

Let that aroma come into your memory now.

Notice how the smell stimulates your taste buds, and your mouth begins to water.

The pleasure of anticipating the sweet taste comes to you before opening the skin.

And now, open the husk of the tangerine but don't eat the fruit yet.

Listen closely to hear the quiet sound of the skin breaking and releasing.

Notice how there is an intense burst of scent,

The pungent perfume fills the air.

Peel the skin back, feeling the strength as the husk releases its fruit.

The vulnerability of the skin as it tears,

The contrast between the white of the inner membranes and the shell.

It is now prepared to offer the nourishment that it contains within.

Vitamin C is one of the most fragile of necessities.

It is water soluble and easily taken into your bloodstream through your saliva.

Your mouth seems to know and to anticipate that process.

Its goodness will become part of you, strengthening your body in ways you may never have thought about.

By bringing its strength to you, you honor the fruit for its power and goodness.

Slowly and deliberately,

Taste the fruit.

Enjoy each segment,

The way the flavor rests on your tongue,

The subtle aftertaste lingers.

Ponder it before you take the next.

As the juice releases itself into your mouth,

Notice the way your salivary glands know just what to do.

Listen again to the tiny sounds of each section breaking apart,

The threads that hold it in place are a network,

To pull it out affects the whole group.

The threads hold each piece in place.

Listen to the sounds within you,

As your tongue moves,

The bursting of juice with the breaking of the membranes.

Notice that process of nutritional absorption as if it is the first time you ever heard, felt, and enjoyed the pleasures of the gift the citrus orchard has given to you.

Take a deep breath and savor the process.

Enjoy each moment.

And now while the sensations are fresh in our minds,

Let us review each of those sensory feelings.

Can you see the beauty of the whole tangerine before you opened it?

The beauty of the irregularities?

The sharp contrasts in color and shape near the stem?

The intense vivid orange and green?

Can you smell the scent of the skin?

How it released its fragrance fully when it was pierced?

The shape and weight of the whole fruit in your hand,

The manner in which the fruit willfully released its tender center,

Now within your belly bringing transformed into a gift of nourishment.

These images are within you, part of you.

How different was the anticipation from the experience?

Can you remember the sense of eagerness?

Can you enjoy that part and how much it added the experience?

How anticipation amplified the experience,

The memory of each step along the way,

Paints itself within your mind's eye,

For you to recall, enjoy, look back upon, and enjoy again and again whenever you want.

Observations

Although the environment for this activity was often noisier than optimal, the participants had little difficulty focusing attention on the tangerine and its sensory elements. The occasional spontaneous comments by group members serve to deepen the experience. If a client is exceedingly distractible and eats her tangerine early, be prepared to go with that. Feedback was overwhelmingly enthusiastic and very positive. Participants were able to embrace the experience and enjoy the activity in self-discipline. Several noted that it was the best tangerine they ever ate in their life, and others noted they had already begun to anticipate going into the lunchroom and selecting another one of the tangerines to repeat the activity on their own.

Inspired by: Childhood exercises.

"Use connections from your creative unconscious to make more connections into the world."

STEPHEN GILLLIGAN

Sensory Treasure Hunt

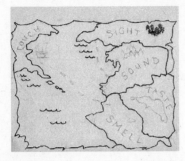

Location: Outdoors

Time: 30–45 minutes

Materials: Sensory Treasure Hunt Handout (one per person)

Pens or pencils

Small prizes (small candies, pens, or other tokens)

Objectives

- To engage the use of all senses.
- To stimulate the senses in the present moment and in the imagination.
- To improve environmental awareness, cognitive stimulation, and communication.

Directions

1. Give participants a Sensory Treasure Hunt Handout and a pen or pencil.
2. Gather group outside and instruct participants to fill out the blanks in the handout.
3. Designate a time and place to meet at the end.
4. Award prizes to each person as he or she completes the sensory treasure hunt.

Observations

This was an activity that got everyone moving around and using all their senses. It would be a good choice to do at an outing at the lake or the park. The group enjoyed sharing their memories. Participants relished the idea of receiving a prize even if it was very small. There is some evidence that for individuals with cognitive impairment, activities using multi-sensory stimulation may improve and increase synaptic connections and neuron-transmission. This activity also intentionally calls upon past sensory memories. For more information, you may look up Snoezelen (developed in the Netherlands), multisensory environment therapies (MSE), or multisensory stimulation techniques.

Inspired by: Scavenger hunts done with friends as a teenager and research on the benefits in rehabilitation of multisensory stimulation.

Sensory Treasure Hunt HANDOUT

Can you find these things?
Write about what you find!
Complete the list and win a prize!

What can you see? Find something:

Orange_____

Yellow _____

Green_____

Blue _____

Purple _____

Brown _____

Round _____

Funny-shaped _____

White_____

Clear _____

Multicolored _____

What can you smell? Find something that smells:

Good _____

Bad _____

Strong _____

What can you hear? Listen for these sounds:

Something in nature _____

People sound_____

Pleasant sound _____

I can barely hear it_____

What can you touch? Look for these textures:

Something smooth _____

Something rough_____

Something hard_____

Something that is itchy _____

Something sharp _____

What about taste? Think about these things:

Name something good you will taste today _____

What does your toothpaste taste like? _____

In your memory or your imagination, think of something:

SIGHT

Wonderful _____

Bright _____

Beautiful _____

Special _____

SMELL

That makes you hungry _____

That makes you calm _____

Fresh _____

A favorite flower _____

SOUNDS

Something pretty from long ago _____

A song in your heart _____

TOUCH

A favorite piece of clothing against your skin _____

Someone who made you smile _____

Something out of reach that you wish you could touch _____

TASTE

A food that you enjoyed in childhood but haven't had for years _____

A food you ate on the last holiday _____

What helps you?

Feel comfortable inside _____

Feel spiritual _____

Feel good to be alive _____

Look forward to tomorrow _____

"Many of the lessons embedded within the exercises are fundamental to success in society."

ROXANNA ERICKSON-KLEIN

Serenity Boxes

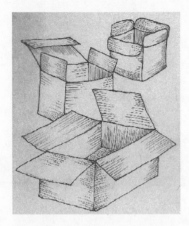

Location: Indoors

Time: 90 minutes

Materials: Small boxes with lids (one per person)

Pencils, colored markers, or small bottles of paint

Colored or patterned craft or scrapbook paper

Magazines for collage

Variety of craft items for decoration (glitter, jewels, letter cutouts, pre-printed recovery slogans)

Glue or glue sticks

Scissors

Objectives

- To teach a productive way to release anxieties, worries, and obsessions.

Directions

1. Before the session, collect small paper or cardboard boxes with lids and materials to decorate the boxes. These can be bought at craft stores or recycled from home, such as empty tea boxes or snack cannisters.

2. Read aloud the concept of a serenity box:
   The idea is to have a box with a slot; it can open or not open. Write your troubles, your wishes, your obsessions, your hard-to-make decisions, or things you are struggling with on a small piece of paper and deposit them in the box. By doing this, you "let go and let God" or "release it to Nature." Symbolically, you really do "let it go."

3. Have participants choose a box from those available.

4. Encourage participants to decorate their box in a meaningful way.

5. Once participants complete their box, read aloud the following benefits of placing worries and troubles in the box:
   What you do with your slips of paper is up to you. Some people choose to leave the notes in the sealed box. Some may choose not to close the box, so periodically the notes can be thrown away without reading them again. Others benefit from looking through the slips of paper periodically before tossing them away or tearing them up, shredding them, or even burning them in a safe place. If you reread them at a later date, you will be surprised to find that most of your worrying was pointless, and the scenarios you imagined at the time never came to pass.

   At the end of the day, take a few minutes to write one or two of your concerns on slips of paper and place them inside the box. Or if the box is handy, you can write worries as each crops up and drop your worries into the box throughout the day.

6. Have each participant present his or her finished box to the group and explain how it will be used.

Observations

Some participants will have done this activity before, and it will be new to others. The box is sometimes called a God box or worry box. Many in early recovery found it a useful coping tool to use when anxieties became overwhelming. Serenity boxes are great for anyone who has trouble with chronic anxiety and encourages turning problems over to a Higher Power. Everyone gets distracted by worries and concerns, but sometimes they can get out of control and interfere with the day. Having a place to literally contain worries may help us set them aside so we can stop obsessing and move forward.

Inspired by: Traditional recovery activity.

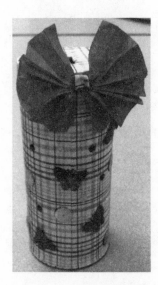
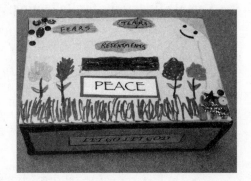

Three Meals

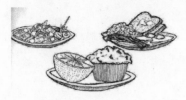

Location: Indoors

Time: 60–90 minutes

Materials: Three Meals Handout (one per person)

Colored construction paper

Pens or markers

Plain paper plates (three per person)

Magazines for collage

Glue

Additional handouts on healthy eating

Objectives

- To conceptualize the process of healthy eating.
- To identify the healthy progression of self-care that has already begun.
- To envision an ongoing ability to continue one's healthy progression.

Directions

1. Find additional handouts on healthy eating. The website for the United States Department of Agriculture is a good source.

2. Pass out Three Meals Handout and provide some basic information about healthy eating.

3. Have an informal discussion about attending to one's own dietary needs.

4. Choose one meal to focus on, such as breakfast, and illustrate:

   - One meal eaten while using substances.
   - One meal eaten in a recovery setting.
   - One meal planned or anticipated in a future healthy time.

5. Encourage participants to reflect upon eating habits they had, have now, and would like to have in the future.

   ### Sample Questions for Reflection:

   - How good of a job am I doing meeting my own nutritional needs?
   - Do I have knowledge about healthy eating?
   - Do I know where to go to learn more?
   - Do I practice good eating habits?
   - Am I a good body weight?
   - Do I have any special restrictions, preferences, or needs?

6. Ask participants to consider whether or not they have adequate knowledge about their own nutritional needs.

7. Instruct participants use the paper plates to decorate samples of their own meals.

8. Allow sufficient time for participants to illustrate their plates and discuss their experiences.

Observations

This activity was done with a group of twenty. Most had an awareness of the fundamentals of healthy eating, including special restrictions such as low salt or low fat. There was also awareness of portion size and of the concept of empty calories. Illustrations of their diets while using substances provided another tool for reflection on the effects of their behavior. The transition into healthier eating reinforced the progress made and the prospect of planning healthy meals seemed to offer a sense of empowerment.

Inspired by: Many inpatients gain weight during treatment and developing awareness and acceptance of responsibility for healthy eating is important.

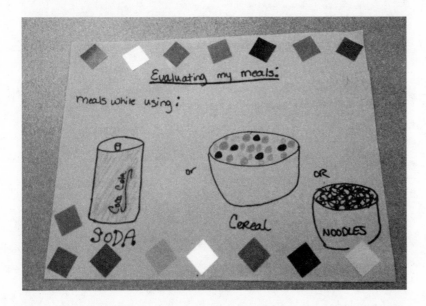

Meals "while using" for this person consisted of soda, cereal, or noodles.

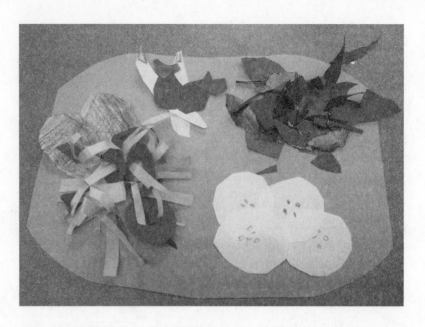

A representation of a balanced meal with vegetables and fruit.

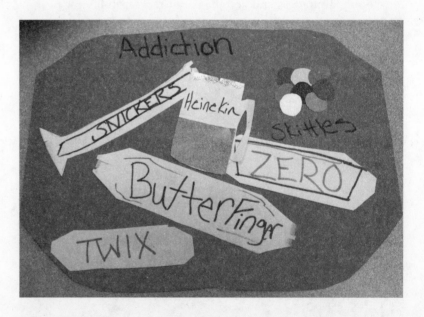

A meal for one person during addiction was candy and beer.

Three Meals HANDOUT

The purpose of this activity is to increase your awareness about dietary habits and to encourage healthy eating.

- Use the paper plates and art supplies to assist in reviewing your own dietary habits.

- Choose breakfast, lunch, or dinner so the comparisons are meaningful.

- Describe a typical meal that you ate while using alcohol or other drugs.

- Describe a meal you are currently eating.

- Describe a meal you think represents a healthy way to eat.

- Using the informational handouts, evaluate your meals for quality, quantity, and overall health.

Quality

- Do the meals contain nutritionally balanced foods?

- Are you now eating a balanced diet containing protein, fresh fruits, and vegetables?

- Do you know what changes you could make to make the meals even healthier?

- Are there some changes that could be made to the future meal to make it healthier, or is it already healthy?

Quantity

- Do you eat enough to give you energy for good performance?

- Are you eating more or less calories than you need?

Overall Health

- Do you believe you have a balanced diet?

- Do you have special needs, such as diabetes or weight loss, to address in your meal evaluation?

- Are there changes you can make now to help you?

- Do you need more guidance or education?

Twelve-Step Scroll

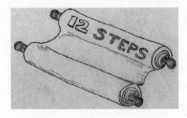

Location: Indoors

Time: 60 minutes

Materials: 12" wooden dowels (two per person)

Roll of paper or gift wrap

Duct or electrical tape

Ribbon

Colored markers

The Twelve Steps (See Appendix. One per person.)

Optional: Beads and other decorations

Objectives
- To explore an unfamiliar way of expressing and displaying valued information.

Directions
1. Before the sesssion, prepare wooden dowels by cutting into twelve-inch lengths. Alternatively, unsharpened pencils can serve as miniature dowels, but this requires smaller paper for display. Paper will be affixed to the dowels, so it may need to be cut for size ahead of time. Gift wrap can be cut in varying lengths and makes an attractive scroll. Provide copies of the Twelve Steps for participants to copy or glue onto their scrolls.

2. Ask participants to choose two dowels and paper that is slightly narrower than the dowels.

3. Instruct participants to attach paper to the top dowel using duct or electrical tape. Then have them repeat with the bottom dowel.

4. Have participants construct a hanging ribbon by affixing it to each end of the top dowel.

5. Tell participants to write the Twelve Steps or other desired contents on the scroll. Participants may cut each Step from the handout and glue it to the paper, if writing is problematic.

6. Have participants decorate the scroll as desired.

7. When participants are done, encourage them to roll up the scroll and tie with ribbon, or hang it on a wall.

8. Ask volunteers to show their scroll and discuss its meaning.

Observations

This activity was done in a group of thirty-four, each of varying ability and functioning. The preference for most participants was to use handouts of the Twelve Steps to cut and glue for display on the scroll. Gluing layers of paper interfered with rolling up of the scrolls, so this proved appropriate for those who wished to hang their scroll. Several people used pencils as dowels and small versions of the Twelve Steps to display. A variety of original designs were created, and the overall reception was very positive. The interest in discussing and showing the work was so great that another group session was set aside for the purpose of discussing the meaning to each participant.

Inspired by: A display of Egyptian papyrus.

Communicating with Others: Expressive Verbal and Nonverbal Connections

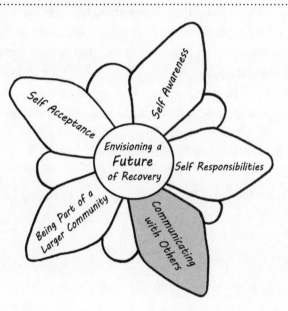

Substance abuse overtakes healthy social functioning in pervasive ways. Dysfunctional relationships can contribute to the addiction cycle, and behavior changes damage healthy relationships. Energy and time become increasingly consumed by addictive activities that limit opportunities for healthy social interactions. Changes in living circumstances, associated with either addiction or recovery, in combination with loss of long-term relationships can leave individuals with a sense of devastation. Support groups can and do provide a bridge to avoid isolation and facilitate reintegration into society. Even with that readily available resource, social limitations can interfere with effective social integration.

Those who start with limited social skills, or who have lost some social graces, will benefit from some basic activities to build skills and get feedback from others. The activities in this section emphasize self-expression and listening to others, as well as attention to nonverbal communication. Also the activities give a platform for recognition of what others are communicating as well as expression in ways that others can understand.

Roxanna: In discussing the process of communication with a group, the concept of nonverbal messages is explored. The participants with a history of prostitution freely shared a sharp acuity to nonverbal signals. Though there may have been a degree of exaggeration, one woman told about a court date in which she had been dropped off at the curb in front of the courthouse. In the twenty-minute interval after being dropped off, she managed to solicit a john, perform services, collect cash, purchase drugs, and take them all before rejoining the driver who had been entrusted to accompany her to court. The volunteer who had inadvertently enabled the relapse was not aware of what had happened, and it was the client who suffered from remorse and called this to the attention of the counselor. As counterproductive as the above actions were, there are several lessons to be learned from this story. Among them is the tremendous capacity for human beings to learn to identify messages from others. Nonjudgmental acceptance of this remarkable admission of a client about her morning activities was effectively reframed into a valuable therapeutic session. Of course, follow-up related with the policies, as well as with the clients plan of care, were implemented.

Kay: Those with addiction often lose basic, human, social connections. Our clients come into treatment with diminished abilities to maintain good social networks, cooperate socially, and have empathy for others. "Active Listening Skills" and "Getting to Know You" were developed to practice simple and appropriate spoken communication with other people. "Magic Hands" promotes positive nonverbal communication with imitation of body movements. In this particular activity, participants may engage their mirror neurons to understand the actions of others and learn by imitation.

"Listen to My Song" was always a favorite activity with my clients. The music never failed to provoke strong feelings and thoughts about past actions and future hopes. The symbolism in the lyrics always held different meanings for various members of the group. Many times, the groups burst into spontaneous singing or dance movements, which created a strong bond of connectivity with others.

Active Listening Skills

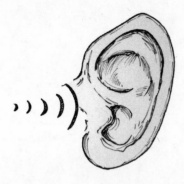

Location: Indoors or Outdoors

Time: 45 minutes

Materials: Active Listening Skills Handout

Objectives

- To teach and practice active listening skills.
- To improve communication skills.

Directions

1. Discuss things that help people communicate well. Misunderstanding is the heart of many arguments and hurt feelings. How does it make us feel when we have people who we can talk to about something important to us? What do we like about that? Ask the group to think about the last time they witnessed others having a conflict. Did the two parties listen to each other well? Or did they interrupt and talk over each other?

2. Distribute the Active Listening Skills Handout and review the Keys to Effective Listening.

3. Have two volunteers demonstrate effective listening and poor listening.

4. Ask everyone to break into pairs and take turns being the talker and the listener. One partner will answer each of the seven questions. The other partner will actively listen.

5. Instruct the partners to switch roles.

6. After switching roles, have a group discussion.

7. Ask participants to take a moment and think about something they learned about their partner. Ask for volunteers to share.

8. Continue the discussion by asking participants how difficult it was to only listen.

9. Encourage volunteers to demonstrate one or two of the questions. You can also ask volunteers to role play NOT using these skills and compare the differences.

Observations

At a residential treatment center, there are daily conflicts and misunderstandings. Deficient social skills and lack of self-awareness can lead to poor communications with others. We found group members open to improving their relationships with others and willing to practice the skills presented in this activity.

Inspired by: A need for enhanced communication within a residential program.

Active Listening Skills HANDOUT

Keys to Effective Listening

- Stop working.

- Stop reading, watching TV, and listening to music.

- Stop texting; put your phone down.

- Look at the other person. Make eye contact.

- Keep a comfortable distance between you and the other person.

- Turn toward other person; uncross arms.

- Think about your facial expressions and try to stay neutral (no rolling eyes, smirking, or frowning).

- Nod your head as the other person talks and make statements such as "uh-huh" or "okay." Use the phrases "I understand" or "I see what you mean" to show the other person you understand what he or she is saying.

- If you don't understand, let the other person know. Ask for clarification. Don't fake it!

- When other person is done speaking, provide a summary of what was said to see if you heard correctly. "Ok, what I hear you saying is . . . "

- Do not make judgments; give advice. Avoid telling other person how you handled something similar. You do not have to provide any answers; you are just listening.

- Be curious and ask questions to show you are interested in what the person is saying.

- Do not interrupt the person speaking.

Active Listening Activity

Instructions: Sit with your partner and take turns being the talker and the listener. First person will answer the questions. The other partner will listen actively. Then switch. Do not take notes. Remember to use the active listening skills we discussed. This should take ten to fifteen minutes. When you are done, please return to the group and be quiet until everyone is finished.

1. When was the first time you got drunk or high?

2. Give three examples of feelings or moods you have tried to change by using alcohol or other drugs?

3. What is your greatest fear about being in recovery?

4. What positive changes would you like to make in your life?

5. If you were a powerful king or queen, what would you do?

6. If someone cooked you a wonderful meal, what would you want on the menu?

7. What would you like to see yourself doing a year from now?

Another View

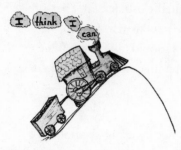

Objectives

- To promote use of imaginary resources to find comfort in the presence of discomfort.

- To teach how small changes in attitude can vastly impact responses and that there are often simple effective ways to deal will issues that arise in recovery.

Directions

1. Sit in a circle so that participants are facing each other.

2. Pass out the Another View Handout containing sentence frames.

3. Explain the rules, parameters, and expectations of the activity.

   - Problems expressed should be small inconveniences, not large or life threatening.

   - Responses are expected to be positive and help solve problems.

   - Responses that include fanciful uses of the imagination are encouraged.

   - Do not spend time searching for a perfect answer; the activity works best when positive energy flows at a rapid pace.

   - Be respectful of the problems expressed and the responses offered.

   - The purpose is to learn to find comfort despite situations that are not so changeable.

4. Ask the first participant to express a complaint, preferably one they have experienced in the current setting. For example, "I don't like group," "I don't like to get up early," or "I'm tired."

5. Ask the participant sitting to the right to respond using the first sentence stem from the handout. For example, "Can you imagine how it would be if . . . we actually learned something useful in group."

6. Instruct the next person in the circle to use the second sentence stem to respond.

Location: Indoors

Time: 25–30 minutes

Materials: Another View Handouts (one per person)

Pencils or pens

Paper

7. Have each group member respond sequentially to the complaint with a positive message.

8. When it is the complainer's turn, the participant to the right expresses a different complaint.

9. Start a second round using the same sequence.

10. After a round or two, relax the format and encourage participants to abandon the sequence and use whatever sentence stem they want.

11. Continue until everyone in the circle has a chance to express a complaint and to listen to all of the suggestions for coping with that complaint.

Observations

This activity has been used in various types of groups with great success. In the recovery setting, it was used with two groups, each of about twenty, which was slightly large to get the fast-paced momentum going that brings enthusiasm. However, the facilitator was able to generate participation that became a high-spirited, supportive group. Complaints expressed had to do with the cloudy weather, boredom, and dislike of the food. All complaints were realistic and common to various members of the group. Responses for the most part were creative and adaptive. A few of the participants showed some negativity, but this quickly became obvious, and the group responded. At times, the sentence stems may not synchronize perfectly with an identified complaint, but participants are encouraged to continue with the spirit of the activity. Comments about meals were answered with sensitive replies, such as "I know someone who doesn't have enough to eat," and with comments that brought laughter, "You might begin to notice that this is a lot better than jail food." A couple of individuals had medical concerns, and their related complaints required appropriate follow-up for assessment and treatment. By the end of the second round, there were numerous comments about how the time spent drastically changed attitudes.

Inspired by: An exercise learned from Stephen Gilligan and Paul Carter.

Another View HANDOUT

Sentence Stems

Use these sentence stems or create your own to begin your response to someone's complaint.

Can you imagine how it would be if . . .

Do you remember the feeling of when . . .

Sometimes, like magic, the sensation can change . . .

The body is marvelous . . .

I knew someone who . . .

You might begin to notice . . .

I wonder when you will start . . .

You might not have noticed yet . . .

What happens when you . . .

Notice the sensation of . . .

Maybe you haven't . . .

You might want to . . .

Sooner or later . . .

I'm wondering if . . .

People can always . . .

A small thing you might do is . . .

When that happens to me I . . .

I like to think about . . .

Later this may feel like . . .

Can the feeling change into . . .

"What is easiest to see is
often overlooked."

MILTON H. ERICKSON

Domino and Recovery

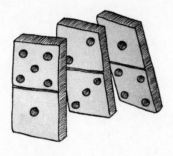

Location: Indoors

Time: 15–30 minutes

Materials: Whiteboard

Dry-erase markers

Objectives

- To enhance positive associations between random items and recovery.

- To strengthen cognitive and communication skills by expressing associations between ideas.

Directions

1. Write the word "domino" on the whiteboard.

2. Pose the following question to the group: "What does a domino have to do with recovery?"

3. Encourage expression of associations that will be useful in recovery. When group members offer ideas, write these ideas on the board.

4. Once five associations have been elicited from the participants, erase the board and invite a volunteer to come to the front and write his or her own random word.

5. Ask the group is to name five associations related to the new word on the board.

6. Rounds continue until each participant offers a random word, and other participants express associations.

Observations

A group of about twenty-five participated in this activity. The initial example of a domino was useful in stimulating participation as various group members wanted to express associations of how one bad choice or one slip can initiate a whole sequence of events. Other associations offered included: "For me it is a trigger as it is a game played in my neighborhood"; "The game involves matching different parts"; and "It's all black and white." Participants caught on quickly, and words offered included: "animal," which generated a great deal of specific and personal imagery, "shoes," "raincloud," and "toy box." While this activity in some ways served as an icebreaker, the intent of the activity goes beyond the immediate conversation to encourage broader self-awareness and coping abilities when random thoughts hit unexpectedly.

Inspired by: Tina Turner's "What's Love Got to Do With It?" written by Terry Britten and Graham Lyle, 1984, Capitol, EMI Music.

Emotional Go Around

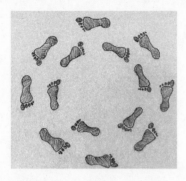

Location: Indoors or Outdoors

Time: 15–25 minutes

Materials: None

Note: You will need a group of 15 or more participants, the larger the better.

Objectives

- To help people identify emotions and body language correctly, both in themselves and others.

- To assist with emotional regulation.

Directions

1. Divide the group in half.

2. Create an interior circle with about half of the group members looking out and an exterior circle with the other group members facing the interior circle. Ask participants to stand at a comfortable distance from one another but keep the circles intact.

3. Explain that the people in the interior circle are the Lookers and the people in the exterior circle are the Actors.

4. Instruct the Actors to make a facial expression that accurately shows their own personal response to the emotion described.

5. Call out **HAPPY** for the first round.

6. Ask the Lookers to note the differences among the ways each person displays his or her emotions.

7. Instruct both circles to walk, one clockwise and one counter clockwise.

8. When the circles return to the starting positions, call out "change roles," and the Lookers become the Actors and vice versa. **HAPPY** is repeated.

9. Another revolution is made.

10. Ask participants to swap roles again and call out another emotion: **SAD**.

11. As the revolutions of the circles continue, provide reminders, such as, "Now the outside circle is the Lookers and the inside circle is the Actors, and the emotion this time is **MAD**."

12. Continue with about ten different emotional expressions.

HAPPY

SAD

MAD

GUILTY

AFRAID

TIRED

ENERGETIC

PLAYFUL

RELAXED

COMFORTABLE

RELIEVED

CURIOUS

REBELLIOUS

THANKFUL

13. When nearing the end of the activity, finish with **THANKFUL**.

14. Wrap up discussion with participants expressing whether they were able to recognize the variations of facial expressions associated with the emotions named.

Observations

This activity was done three times, once with a group of forty-five, once with a group of twenty, and again with another group of seventeen. The first two times the groups had mixed abilities and self-awareness, and the third time it was done with a higher functioning group. The first two times, the activity was well-received with amazing energy produced by the excitement of the activity. The third time, in a higher functioning group, members were more cognitively self-aware and self-responsible, and the activity was not as valuable to them. In the larger group, much appreciation was expressed regarding the opportunity to "see" emotion on the face of twenty other individuals. In one of the sessions, we used a large class setting, and the circles revolved around an exterior pathway. Although the individuals came into contact with each other for only for a portion of the time while they moved, the setting provided even more animation from the group.

This activity is particularly valuable for those group members who have been consumed with addiction. The discussion revealed that many participants are weak in their abilities to either express or interpret facial expressions. Also many participants asked for specific feedback regarding how others responded to their own acting.

Inspired by: In an anger management group activity, it became apparent that some of the group members were having trouble identifying facial expressions of others. This activity was constructed to deal with that concern. The research of Paul Ekman, PhD, on recognition of expression was inspirational, although this is not based directly from his work.

"At times, group members are reluctant to speak words, but creative expression opens additional doors."

KAY COLBERT

Exploring Emotions

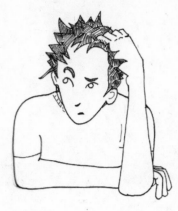

Objectives

- To connect with basic emotions.
- To become aware of verbal and nonverbal manners in which emotions are perceived and acted upon.

Directions

1. Count off to create six groups and pass out the Exploring Emotions Handout.

2. Give each group a card that describes one basic emotion. Groups should refrain from sharing their assigned emotion.

    FEAR Fright, panic, anxiety, dread, worry, distress

    LOVE Affection, longing, caring, tenderness, sentimentality

    SURPRISE Amazement, shock, astonishment

    ANGER Irritation, rage, frustration, resentment, contempt

    SADNESS Sorrow, shame, remorse, guilt, neglect, woe, misery

    JOY Happy, pleasure, contentment, enthusiasm, delight

3. Each group must display the assigned emotion in a series of ways with each group member participating in one or more of the displays.

4. Before beginning, demonstrate the activity. Boredom can be used as an example of an emotion that does not compete with the assigned emotions.

5. Each group must show all four of these displays. Allow for fifteen minutes of consultation time within groups.

    - Still Life: Without words or sounds, use group member(s) to show the emotion through a "look."

Location: Indoors or Outdoors (any area that a stage can be used or imagined)

Time: 45 minutes

Materials: Exploring Emotions Handout (one per person)

Index cards listing one of the basic emotions

- Movie: Without words or sounds, use group member(s) to show the emotion through gestures or actions.

- Sounds: Without words, use vocal tones to express the emotion.

- Description: Using words alone, dictionary style, express the meaning of the emotion, without using the actual name of the emotion.

6. After a group has expressed all four of the displays, the audience guesses which emotion has been displayed.

7. On conclusion of all performances, open group discussion to reflect upon learning.

Observations

This activity took place in an outdoor setting and in an auditorium with a group of about twenty-five women and one facilitator. It was well received and generated active, enthusiastic participation. The facilitator found it more difficult to engage the participants in a discussion inside the auditorium, rather than when they were able to face each other outside. This activity was created after reading a variety of approaches to discussing emotions. It was surprising how little consensus existed.

Inspired by: A multitude of activities in books; therapeutic games that discuss emotions fundamental to human nature.

Exploring Emotions HANDOUT

Note: Do NOT show your assignments to anyone outside of your group. This activity is intended to be a game, and everyone needs to guess which emotion is being acted.

Meet with your group and plan how to present the emotion you are assigned.

- **Still Life:** Without words or sounds, use group members to show emotion through a "look."

- **Movie:** Without words or sounds, use group members to show emotion through gestures or actions.

- **Sounds:** Without words use vocal tones to express emotion.

- **Description:** Using words alone, dictionary style, express the meaning of the emotion without using the name of the emotion.

Each group member needs to participate in one or more of these performances.

You will have fifteen minutes to prepare all of these performances.

Each group will take turns presenting their emotion.

Hold your guesses until the conclusion of each group.

"Many people automatically dismiss their own originality as worthless since it has never been reinforced in their early life experience."

ERNEST ROSSI

Getting to Know You

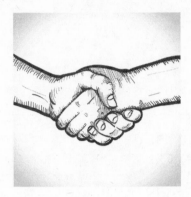

Location: Indoors or Outdoors

Time: 30 minutes

Materials: Pens

Paper

Optional list of questions

Objectives

- To become familiar with others in the group.

- To become aware of specific personal values that can influence choices in making friends.

Directions

To avoid confusion, it may be useful to do a short demonstration with volunteers prior to beginning the activity.

1. Hold a group discussion about the meaning of friendship, which includes trusting one another and the process of finding a network of others with whom one can enjoy spending time.

2. Each participant writes a short question on a piece of paper that reflects some important value. For example: Where do you go to church? How do you like to have fun on the weekend? Have you ever been to a twelve-step meeting?

3. Participant approaches another group member and asks his or her question.

4. The respondent answers with a short reply, offering no additional conversation.

5. Ask the questioner and respondent to switch roles so another question can be asked and replied to.

6. Then participants swap partners and ask their value question to a new partner.

7. Continue until each participant has asked his or her question to at least five others.

8. Ask participants to share their value questions and how the replies they received influenced their feelings about the potential for friendship with each person with whom they spoke.

Observations

This activity was performed twice, once in a recovery setting with twenty-three women and once in a community college setting with twenty-seven freshmen students. In each setting, the tendency to keep talking was challenging for the facilitator to monitor. On both occasions, the participants moved freely through the groups and conversed with others who were outside of their normal range of contact. The questioning phase went rapidly, lasting about ten minutes, but the discussion regarding thoughtful selection of their value question was quite lengthy. In the college setting, students reported later that the activity had made a substantial social impact, particularly among the English as a second language students.

The activity in the recovery setting was well-received. People in recovery revealed anxiety over approaching others and being accepted by those they didn't know well. Clients in recovery often had difficulty making connections with others.

Inspired by: An overheard conversation: "I don't want to ask friends to go to the movies because they might want to go out drinking afterward."

Inspirational Hands

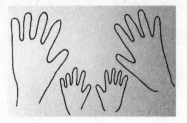

Location: Indoors

Time: 30 minutes

Materials: Paper 8½" × 11" or larger

Markers of various colors

Optional: A copy of inspirational affirmations (See Affirmations in Appendix.)

Objectives

- To provide participants the opportunity to identify positive attributes about themselves.

- To receive feedback from others about how they are received by others.

Directions

1. Ask participants to take one sheet of paper.

2. Instruct participants to trace one hand on one half of the paper.

3. Have participants trace their other hand in the remaining space, asking for help from a fellow participant.

4. On each finger of the left hand, direct participants to list qualities they like about themselves.

5. For the right hand, tell participants to ask another group member to write an adjective that describes what they like about the participant. This should be continued until five different people are asked.

6. Once all ten of fingers have a descriptor of the participant's personal qualities, instruct participant to choose a positive affirmation to write on the paper.

7. Encourage participants to decorate the rest of the picture as desired.

8. Once finished, discuss which qualities listed by other group members surprised them.

Observations

This activity was performed twice, once in a group of ten and a second time in a larger group of twenty-five. Each time, it was well received and deeply appreciated. Many participants were surprised by the adjectives others wrote to describe them. The participants also enjoyed having extra time to decorate the images.

Inspired by: An exercise already in use at Nexus Recovery Center in Dallas, Texas, and therapeutic activities at other centers.

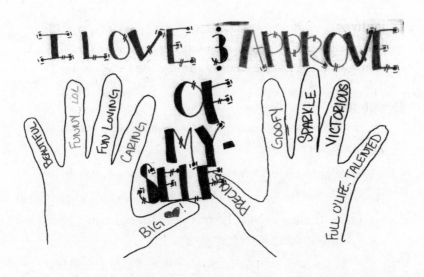

Sample Inspirational Hands titled, "I Love & Approve of Myself,"
celebrating ten positive personal qualities: "Beautiful, Funny LOL,
Fun Loving, Caring, Big Heart, Precious, Goofy, Sparkle, Victorious,
Full o' Life, and Talented."

Lean My Way

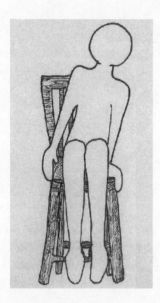

Location: Indoors or Outdoors

Time: 10–15 minutes

Materials: Straight back chair for each participant

Objectives

- To enhance self-awareness through exploration of the ways we make muscle movements without realizing we are doing them.

Directions

1. Begin with a two-minute demonstration with the facilitator and two volunteers.

   - Volunteers decide who will be the Thinker and who will be the Looker.

   - The Thinker and the Looker sit about eighteen inches apart, looking at one another.

   - Without speaking, the Thinker thinks about bending forward or leaning to right or left, but does NOT actually move.

   - The Looker uses a hand signal to indicate which direction he or she believes the Thinker is thinking.

   - When the Looker correctly identifies the direction, the Thinker nods and begins thinking about another movement.

   - After a few rounds swap roles.

2. Ask participants to find a partner.

3. Have participants discuss who will be the Thinker and the Looker.

4. The partners proceed with the activity, without speaking. The Looker uses hand gestures to indicate perceived direction, and the Thinker nods when the guess is correct.

5. After the Looker is able to correctly identify the direction of the Thinker four times in a row, they should swap roles. If this does not evolve in a timely manner, ask them to switch after a few minutes.

6. Open the floor to feedback about the activity.

Observations

This activity was performed dozens of times in various settings with groups ranging in size from ten to fifty participants. The first time this activity was performed, two volunteers demonstrated in front of the larger group, and then others were invited to participate in the second round. Typically after viewing the activity, there was a wholehearted response. It was surprising how quickly all of the participants became tuned in to the small muscle movements that revealed which direction the Thinker was thinking.

Those who observed, but did not participate, were invited to share in the discussion. Within the discussion, some participants said they were apprehensive about being looked at, especially as they did not understand how the Looker was picking up the small signals. Overall, the activity was uncomfortable for some, and leaving it as voluntary was a wise choice. Subsequent sessions in which more preparation time was spent in explaining the body language signals that one "broadcasts" was useful in preparing the participants and led to a higher participation rate. The underlying idea of how this activity pertains to recovery was readily understood, and the activity led to a fertile discussion.

Inspired by: An activity adapted from Maite Garcia, Director, Instituto Ericksoniano de Madrid.

Listen to My Song

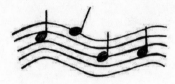

Location: Indoors

Time: 60–90 minutes

Materials: Device that can play pre-selected music

Speakers to play music

Printed song lyrics (one copy per person)

Objectives

- To provide a safe environment for participants to express feelings of anxiety or frustration.

- To support feelings of self-confidence and security and to promote connection with others.

- To demonstrate music can support ongoing success in recovery.

Directions

1. A day or two before the activity, ask participants to pick a song that is meaningful to them in their recovery. Have participants give the name of the song and the name of the artist or group who performs it. This is important as some versions of songs vary greatly.

2. Download each song and print the lyrics. There are several online sites that will provide lyrics at no cost.

3. Make copies of the lyrics for each participant.

4. Instruct each participant to pass out his or her song lyrics before the song is played.

5. Ask each participant if he or she would like to talk about the meaning of the words before or after the piece is played.

6. Take turns playing each participant's song while everyone reads along silently.

7. After each song is played, elicit comments and feelings from others in the group.

Observations

This activity was done at least a dozen times and never failed to elicit strong emotional reactions. It was one of the activities clients enjoyed the most in process group. The activity works best with approximately six to eight clients and also with people who have gotten to know each other. Many times participants wept while listening or explaining their songs. Often, group members asked for a particularly moving song to be replayed at the end, if time allowed.

In one group, there was a young woman with severe depression who had barely spoken since she entered treatment, had a restricted affect, and did not make eye contact. During this activity, she spontaneously began singing to the music in a beautiful voice and then cried when she was finished. This experience provided a natural turning point for her and she was able to open up and share more after that.

When this activity is done with adolescents, it is slightly more challenging. Clear instructions have to be given about the songs they can choose. With this age group, it works best to limit the choices to songs without violent language or cursing. Adolescents need more explanation of how to pick their songs, as well as a reminder that this is not just a chance to listen to music they like, but rather a time to share pieces that have meaning for them in their recovery journey.

Inspired by: A similar activity at another treatment center.

Magic Hands

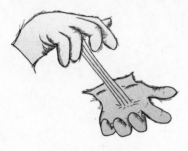

Location: Indoors or Outdoors (Select a space adequate for participants to move around in pairs without bumping into each other.)

Time: 30 minutes

Materials: None

Objectives

- To heighten awareness of nonverbal signals and personal patterns of approach and avoidance in a nonthreatening and friendly atmosphere.

Directions

There are three variations of magic hands. The facilitator and a volunteer demonstrate the different variations and invite group participants to explore the different expressions. Participants are encouraged to notice their awareness and their emotional response to playing and to discuss these aspects with the larger group. General instructions include the idea that the responsibility to remain connected belongs to both the Leader and the Follower and that motions should be smooth, slow, and reasonable. **This is a nonverbal partner activity**.

Hand to Face

1. One person is the Leader, and the other person is the Follower. The partners imagine that the Leader's hand is magnetic and has the power to move the Follower into a position.

2. The leader places his or her palm about six inches from the Follower's face.

3. Ask the leader to slowly move his or her hand from side to side until a connection is felt, maintaining a six-inch gap.

4. The Leader moves around forcing the Follower to reposition, walk around, kneel, or bend into a variety of silly positions.

5. Continue for three minutes.

6. Swap roles.

Mirror Hands

1. One partner is the Leader, and the other partner is the Follower.

2. Partners face one another with both palms facing partner's hands, about six inches apart.

3. Slowly moving his or her hands, the Follower copies the Leader's movements until the relationship is felt, maintaining the six-inch gap.

4. The Leader directs the Follower to move, bend, or reposition for an interval of three minutes.

5. Swap roles.

Four Hands, Push and Pull

1. Partners are both the Leader and the Follower.

2. Partners begin with palms facing one another, about six inches apart.

3. Ask partners to slowly move, maintaining the six-inch gap, until the relationship is felt.

4. Partners "duel" to seek leadership.

5. The Leader "pushes" the partner backward into uncomfortable positions until the partner resists sufficiently to become the Leader.

6. Continue for three minutes or until each participant has experienced both the Leader and the Follower roles.

Observations

These activities were performed with a group of twenty-six, and again with a group of thirty-six women. The demonstration by the group facilitator was crucial for participants to understand expectations. Good natured competition ensued, and active self-reflection about who was a "pushover" and who had "bossy hands" occurred. The group of participants grimaced and made unpleasant facial expressions in efforts to intimidate partners, and on conclusion called out for two of the more creative players to go against one another. Several reported feeling that the activity created awareness of habitual patterns of response as well as attunement to smaller factors such as body space. Several group members with physical limitations participated successfully in a modified version using chairs. This activity encouraged mindfulness and awareness of others and proved to be an excellent way for trauma victims to begin to build trust.

Inspired by: This activity is a variation of a theater-game exercise called "Columbian Hypnosis," described in *Games for Actors and Non-Actors,* 2nd Edition, by Augusto Boal, 1992, Routledge Publishers, New York. This text is an excellent resource for creative movement activities.

"Creative expression goes far beyond what we understand with our conscious minds."

DR. KRISTINA ERICKSON

Masks We Wear

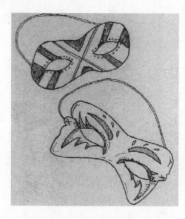

Location: Indoors

Time: 90 minutes

Materials: Mask Templates

Scissors

Glue

Colored pens or paint

Decorative items such as glitter, feathers, or collage materials

Wood craft sticks

Objectives

- To raise awareness about personal patterns of presentation, i.e, what is shown to others and what is kept hidden, sometimes even from the self.

Directions

1. Read the following directions aloud.

   - *On the front of the mask, draw your public face—how you present yourself to most people every day. This is the side that people see including how we want people to view us (our "reputation") and how people label us. When most people think of us, this is what we believe they see.*

   - *On the back of the mask, draw your private face; the face you don't show to everyone. This is who we really are— the aspects of our lives that many people don't know. This is the opportunity to be honest about things that most people may not know about us—past experiences that have formed us, family history, hobbies, interests, hopes, feelings, and dreams.*

2. Remind participants that the mask does not need any facial features drawn or attached, only symbols and words covering both the front and back of the mask.

3. Have participants cut out their masks and glue them on a wood craft stick.

Observations

This activity was performed in a cafeteria setting with a variety of art materials and was embraced seriously. Only a few of the participants showed their private faces to the larger group, although several described their private side. The group was started by a reading a poem about masks and faces.

Inspired by: Decorate-your-own masks at many craft stores.

Masks We Wear TEMPLATE

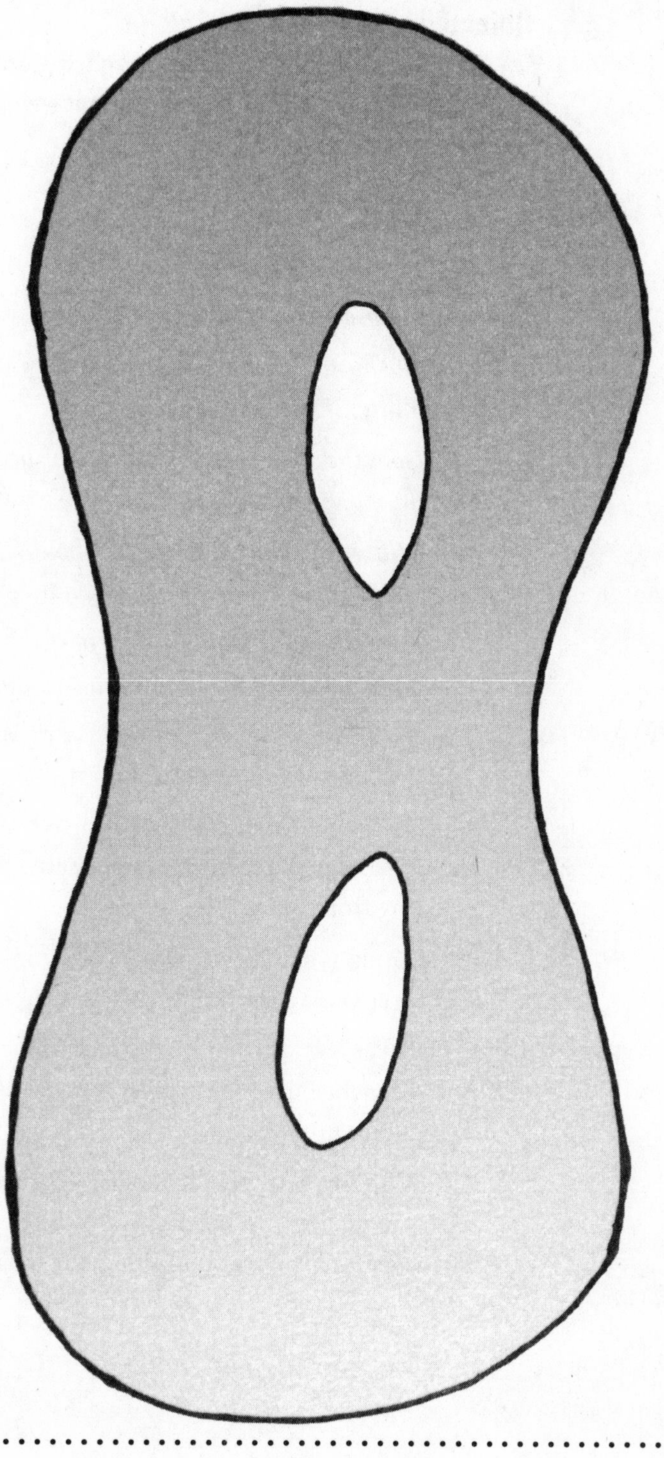

Pendulum Swing

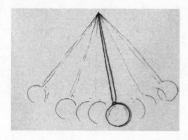

Location: Indoors

Time: 15 minutes

Materials:
For each participant:

A large button, heavy bead or several standard plastic beads

A piece of light string or dental floss about 20"

Timer (clock hand or stopwatch)

Objectives
- To enhance self-awareness through exploration of the ways that we make muscle movements without even knowing that we are doing them.

Directions
1. Read aloud the following instructions.

   - *Choose a bead or button.*

   - *The button or bead is threaded on a string. It does not matter if the string is tied.*

   - *Hold the string with the button or bead between your thumb and forefinger.*

   - *With your hand at eye level, about 18 inches in front of you, dangle the string like a pendulum.*

   - *Keeping your hand and arm perfectly still, close your eyes and IMAGINE the pendulum swinging from left to right.*

   - *After I time you for a minute, open your eyes to see whether or not the pendulum is swinging.*

2. Repeat the activity by asking the participants to keep their arm still and with closed eyes to imagine that the pendulum is swinging front to back, if desired.

3. If the group is sufficiently patient, and time permits, the activity can be repeated a third time. While keeping the arm still, imagine that the pendulum is swinging in a circular motion.

4. At the conclusion of the activity, take a tally of how many saw the pendulum moving when they opened their eyes.

5. Following this activity, encourage a discussion of how this relates to recovery. What body movements are others seeing when we think we are controlling our muscles?

Observations

This activity has been done in a variety of group settings. Typically, about 80 percent of participants find the pendulum swings in the imagined direction. The activity was explained and demonstrated, and participants had a short interval to get ready before they were timed for one minute. The first time we did the activity outdoors with buttons, but the wind interfered. The second time the activity took place indoors with four to six small beads to create the sufficient weight. Although the group was around thirty-five people and participation was voluntary, twenty-one participants did the activity. Fourteen were surprised by seeing the movement in the pendulum, and seven were able to keep the pendulum motionless. The participants were allowed to keep the string and beads and encouraged to use them to stimulate their own curiosity.

Inspired by: As a child, Roxanna's parents allowed her to play with a Ouija board only after careful explanations of the micromuscle movements involved.

Remember Me

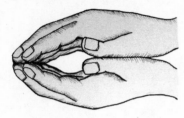

Location: Indoors or Outdoors

Time: 15–30 minutes depending on number of participants

Materials: None

Objectives

- To improve focus and sustained attention skills.
- To recognize positive attributes in oneself.
- To enhance communication skills.

Directions

1. Have participants stand in a circle. Read aloud the following instructions.

   One at a time, introduce yourself using your first name.

   Make a physical gesture (hand clap, turning around, hopping on one foot, or something similar).

   Say one POSITIVE thing about yourself.

2. Provide an example, such as "I am Jenny (clap), and I am generous to others."

3. Explain to participants that the next person has to do the same thing, but also repeat Jenny's name and gesture.

4. Go around the circle until each person is introduced. As it will get increasingly difficult, participants may prompt each other.

Observations

This is a good warm-up activity for a group. Participants had to pay close attention to each other and use their memory skills. Some people found this much easier than others, but it induced good-natured laughter when difficulties arose. When used in a group of approximately ten, participants were able to recall names. In larger groups, prompting by others helped the activity. This activity promoted increased familiarity, movement, and laughter.

Inspired by: A similar icebreaker activity done by a staff member at a workshop.

"... it is essential to surround yourself with a community of open hands who believe in you more than you believe in yourself."

PATRICK CARNES

Sensory Match Up

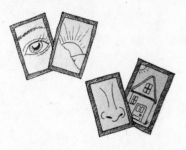

Location: Indoors or Outdoors

Time: 10–15 minutes

Materials: Sensory Match Up Handout (copied on different colored paper and cut into strips)

Objectives

- To stimulate the imaginative process of engaging sensory modalities in different times and locations.

- To increase sensory self-awareness.

Directions

1. Copy the Sensory Match Up Handout on two different colors of paper and cut into strips. One color is for the time or circumstance stems, and the other is for the sensory or physical stems. It is useful to have four volunteers demonstrate and show the process of sharing and then swapping colors.

2. Hand out one strip to each participant. There should be an equal number of each of the two colors.

3. Ask for two volunteers, each with a different colored strip.

   Sample sentences:
   I remember <u>seeing</u> a beautiful sunrise.
   I remember <u>seeing</u> the grass outside.
   I imagine <u>smelling</u> soap when I washed this morning.
   I imagine <u>smelling</u> flowers.
   Just out of reach, there is <u>movement</u>.
   Just out of reach, <u>I move</u> closer to what I want.

4. Tell participants to make an original sentence from the two stems.

5. When done sharing their sentences, ask the participants to swap strips, so they have the other color.

6. Direct participants to roam and select a new partner with the opposite color.

7. Repeat with the entire group for four or five rounds.

Observations

This activity works well in large groups. It is brief and allows participants to mingle. Some are very adept at creatively constructing images, while others struggle with the concept. The fragments do not always come together exactly right, but the challenge invites flexibility in thinking. Each time this activity was done, participants found it was unexpectedly helpful in bringing shy or isolated members into the group.

Inspired by: A variation on a children's get acquainted game.

Sensory Match Up HANDOUT

Sensory Stem: Time or circumstance
Cut the following into individual strips. • Copy on colored paper.

I remember

I imagine

Around me now

Outside of this room

Somewhere in this building

I dream at night about

I daydream about

It is pleasant for me

Long ago

Sometime next year

Happens without noticing

Feels really good when I notice

Suddenly I realize

Happens to someone around me

Wish I could

Notice far away

Notice a change

Seems quick

Lingers for a while

Sometime today

Sometime yesterday

Sometime tomorrow

Would like to more often

Just out of reach

Just now

In the future

I hope for

I look forward to

In the past

Someone else

Sensory Stem: Sensory or Physical • Copy on contrasting colored paper

See

Smell

Taste

Feel texture

Body position

Feel temperature

Feel pressure

Feel light touch

Movement

Feel body stretch

Breathe

Yawn

Hiccup

Tense muscles

Relax muscles

Chew

Close eyes

Touch with fingers

Feel on skin

Close my hand

Describe in words

Get a mental picture

Enjoy the colors

Feel the support of

Mouth waters

Position in the room

Think About Me

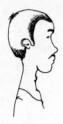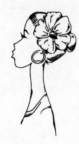

Objectives

- To become more aware of nonverbal, subtle messages that are part of communication.

Directions

1. Begin with a two-minute demonstration with the facilitator and two volunteers.

   - Identify the volunteers as the Thinker and the Looker.

   - Complete the demonstration in short intervals (about fifteen seconds) so the audience can get an understanding of the expectations.

   - Instruct the Thinker and the Looker to gaze steadily and silently into one another's eyes, sitting or standing about three feet apart.

   - In the first timed round, ask the Thinker to *think* one of the following topics:

     a. *You (the Looker) are wonderful.*

     You're so wonderful: looking at the person sitting across, notice as many things that are good about that person, such as eye color, nice hair, sweet personality, or pleasant voice.

     OR

     b. Some random thought, such as, *I have laundry to do.*

     Random thoughts: grocery list, paying bills, daily routine, what's for lunch?

   - Time for fifteen seconds and then say, "Relax your eyes, but don't speak."

   - After a brief pause, initiate the second round, and say to the Thinker, "Change topics—whatever you thought about before, now think the other."

Location: Indoors or Outdoors

Time: 10–15 minutes

Materials: A clock with a second hand

Timer

Bell or chime

- During the third round, instruct the volunteers to swap roles: The Thinker becomes the Looker, and the Looker becomes the Thinker.

- Repeat the third and fourth timed rounds with no discussion.

- At the conclusion of the fourth round, ask the volunteers to identify whether or not they could distinguish whether the partner was "thinking about me" or some random topic.

2. Instruct the remainder of the group to find a partner and agree who will be the Thinker and the Looker for the first two rounds.

3. Remind participants to not speak until the complete activity has concluded. Add that each round will last thirty seconds.

4. Begin round one: Thinker chooses to think "Random Thoughts" or "You're So Wonderful" thoughts.

5. After thirty seconds, announce the end of round one, and remind everone to remain silent.

6. Begin round two: Instruct the Thinker to change topics.

7. Begin round three: Instruct the participants to swap the roles of the Thinker and the Looker.

8. Begin round four: Direct the (new) Thinker to change topics.

9. When time is up, invite the group to confer with partners and guess whether it was in the first or in the second round that the Thinker was "thinking about me."

10. Afterward, provide group members with the opportunity to confer with their partners.

11. Tally the accuracy of the group as a whole.

Observations

This activity was performed with four varying groups. In each case, the participants were given the choice to opt out but still needed to observe the others. In the first large group of about fifty, it appeared there were approximately 60 percent who correctly identified the action of the Thinker. A second group with only ten participants had 100 percent success rate. The third time it was conducted with a group of twenty-four participants and a dozen opted out but watched. Participants again came up with two-thirds correctly identifying the Thinker's thoughts. The fourth try, with a group of twenty participants and a dozen or more watchers, resulted in a 95 percent success rate in correctly recognizing the Thinker's thoughts. The participants, as well as the facilitators, were surprised with the accuracy which is beyond statistical probability.

Inspired by: A group activity learned from Betty Alice Erickson, LPC.

"Learning from one another is a profoundly powerful tool that we call forward in the service of recovery."

Roxanna Erickson-Klein

Twelve Steps to Recovery

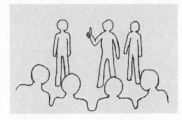

Location: Indoors or Outdoors (need space for participants to present in front of group)

Time: 90 minutes

Materials: Copies of the Twelve Steps for each participant (The Alcoholics Anonymous and Narcotics Anonymous Twelve Steps are provided in the Appendix, but you can use other versions as appropriate.)

Objectives

- To familiarize participants with the Twelve Steps.
- To encourage taking time to deconstruct each Step and interpret the Steps in a personal and meaningful way.

Directions

1. Hand out copies of the Twelve Steps to participants.
2. Instruct participants to form groups of four people.
3. Depending on the number of groups, assign one or more of the Steps for them to present.
4. Allow approximately fifteen minutes for planning.
5. Direct each group to present sequentially in the front of the room. Then ask each group to read aloud the Step(s) and act out what the Step means or looks like to them.

Observations

This activity encouraged participants in residential treatment to stop and think about what each Step really says and what meaning it has for them personally. This was activity completed four times and worked as well for a very large group as it did for a smaller one. With large groups, the teams can present a single step, while smaller groups may have their teams present several steps. This activity also promotes cooperation and planning with others.

Alternative versions of the Twelve Steps can also promote interesting discussions. These variations might include NA, HA, CA, MA, GA, CODA, Zen Twelve Steps, Yes Twelve Steps, Women for Sobriety Thirteen Affirmations, Buddhist Non-theistic Twelve Steps, the Sixteen Steps, or Humanist Twelve Steps. On occasion, participants will say they do not believe in a Higher Power or they feel the Twelve Steps are too old fashioned or have some other reason why they "can't" participate in the activity. Presenting alternative versions of the Steps can often draw in these reluctant members.

Inspired by: Propensity of individuals to interpret each Step in a way that is personally meaningful.

"Healing the wounds of the past is possible. Creating a life worth living is possible. Recovery is possible."

KAY COLBERT

You Tell Me, Then Tell Us

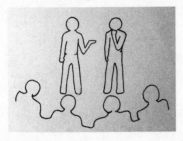

Location: Indoors

Time: 60 minutes

Materials: Pen

Paper

You Tell Me, You Tell Us
Handout (two copies)

Objectives

- To get in touch with individual needs and learn to express those needs appropriately.

- To enhance acceptance of problem solving advice in a healthy way.

- To stimulate a self-search of healthier alternatives to habitual behaviors.

Directions

1. Ask two volunteers to read aloud the mock-up script on the You Tell Me, You Tell Us Handout so the rest of the group has some clarity on what is expected in the breakout session.

2. Instruct the same volunteers to proceed with the Group Report.

3. Answer questions about what is to be done in the breakout sessions and in the activity as a whole. The goal is to generate possible solutions to one's own problems.

4. Direct participants to find a partner. It is unimportant whether pairs include friends or new acquaintances.

5. Spend fifteen minutes in breakout groups in which the following action is taken:

   - Each partner thinks up a small problem that he or she is having some annoyance with, something they don't mind sharing with the group. The problem can be a topic, such as "annoyed by schedule," "don't like the food," "asked to do things that don't seem comfortable," or "have trouble falling asleep."

   - Individually, each partner thinks about his or her own problem and writes a brief description of the problem. Once partners have described their problems in writing, one becomes the Complainer and the partner becomes the Listener.

   - The Complainer tells his or her problem.

- The Listener responds with questions, such as "What might help you to adapt to or change the problem?"

- The Complainer can come up with three possible solutions to help with the problem.

- The Listener writes down three potential alternative, adaptive responses to the problem.

- Partners swap roles.

6. Upon reconvening, ask the pairs to present the problems to the group in a systematic sequence or volunteer basis.

7. As time allows, encourage group discussion of solutions.

Observations

This activity was performed with a group of twenty-eight participants and one facilitator. The group started and ended the breakout sessions with productive conversations. A few of the participants refused to pair up and were individually approached during the breakout interval by the facilitator. They were permissively encouraged to consider the ways in which the activity could be done individually. Surprisingly, each of these participants reported to the group as their turn came, and each person had done effective problem solving. Most of the problems presented included frustrations related to limitations and conditions of the facility: not enough smoke breaks, not enough free time, roommate snores, or not enough phone time. Other concerns addressed included feeling overwhelmed and uncertain about future needs: making living arrangements, getting a social security card, or refilling medications. A few concerns related directly to recovery including anticipation of being exposed to triggers and uncertainties about forming a new friendship group. In all but a few cases, the participants were able to come up with three appropriate, adaptive, and effective ways to solve problems using their own internal creative thinking. Some participants leaned more heavily on their partners than others but for the most part, changes in behavior or attitude seemed to be internally driven. In the few cases in which the participants requested help, other group members were ready to offer appropriate, adaptive adjustments. In only one case did a participant use the forum to express frustrations rather than seek solutions. The step of having the Complainer briefly write a description of the problem effectively minimizes unproductive, descriptive rehashing of the problem phase. Overall, the session was both creative and productive.

Inspired by: This self-directed adaptation activity was inspired by the Cognitive Behavioral Therapy strategies of Christine Padesky, and the Solution Focused approaches taught by Insoo Kim Berg.

You Tell Me, Then Tell Us HANDOUT

BEGIN MOCK UP

Listener Tell me what you would like to work on.

Complainer I guess I could work on not being able to go to sleep at night.

Listener Tell me a little more about that.

Complainer We go to bed here too early for me. Then I have trouble falling asleep. Then I get angry at the schedule. So I try to get the night staff to let me stay up later.

Listener What can you do to change this from happening?

Complainer Maybe I could pretend that it's midnight even though it's only 9 p.m.

Listener That sounds good, can you think of something else?

Complainer I can't think of anything else. If I could it wouldn't be a problem.

Listener Keep thinking, there must be something you can do to help you feel sleepy.

Complainer I just keep thinking that this is stupid; I shouldn't have to adjust my sleep schedule.

Listener While you're here, think about the things that YOU can do to adapt to the situation.

Complainer Maybe I can think about songs that I like to listen to and sing myself to sleep.

Listener That's good, if you don't wake up your roommate.

Complainer I can sing to myself in my head.

Listener That's good then. You've got two. Let's find a third one.

Complainer Maybe I could take a hot shower before I go to bed, that sometimes helps me.

Listener Great work. You did it! You came up with three adaptive solutions.

Complainer Now it's your turn.

SWAP ROLES

Complainer Well, my problem is that I decided to quit smoking when I came here. Every time people talk about smoke breaks, I feel the desire to smoke. Maybe I am trying to make too many changes at once.

Listener Tell me more about the feelings that aren't comfortable.

Complainer I hear the ladies talking about the next smoke break. Then I get angry with myself for choosing this time to quit. I thought I was doing a good thing for myself, but maybe I was being stupid.

Listener What can you do to adapt to the situation here?

Complainer I guess I could recognize that everyone else didn't choose to quit smoking when I did.

Listener That's a start. Does it make you feel better?

Complainer A little.

Listener What else can you do?

Complainer I really need to plan something good while everyone else is out there smoking.

Listener Something good . . . like what?

Complainer I don't know, maybe doing a little exercise or breathing in some fresh air.

Listener Would that help?

Complainer Maybe. I haven't been to the serenity garden yet.

Listener OK, so far you've told me that you can think about your own choice being separate from everyone else and maybe going to the serenity garden. That's two. Can you come up with a third one?

Complainer I could do some stretching exercises. That might make a difference. I haven't tried it.

Listener Great. You have three.

GROUP REPORT

First partner: My problem is I don't usually go to bed so early. I get annoyed at having to go to bed early here. I have trouble falling asleep. The changes in my thinking and behavior I came up with are:

- I can pretend it's midnight when it's really 9 p.m.
- I can try silently singing myself to sleep.
- I can plan to take a hot shower just before it's time to go to bed.

Second partner: My problem is I decided to give up smoking when I came here. Now I'm wondering whether it is a good choice because I feel really bad when everyone else goes off to smoke. The changes in my thinking and behavior I came up with are:

- I can think about the fact that I am making a healthy choice, and it doesn't have anything to do with whether others make the choice to give up smoking or not.
- I can go to the serenity garden for fresh air.
- I can try some stretching exercises every time a smoke break comes up.

"The healthy interaction among group members goes far beyond the moment."

ROXANNA ERICKSON-KLEIN

Being Part of a Larger Community: Participation and Developing a Sense of Belonging

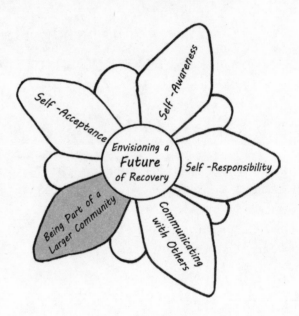

Building a sense of community belonging is as essential as finding meaning in life. Support groups offer a safety net and can prevent social isolation. The generation of new possibilities will serve to bolster support in an ongoing way. The activities in this section are designed to educate individuals about finding and using resources that are accessible, which can enhance success. They serve to increase a sense of meaning, belonging, and resourcefulness.

Often in the interest of recovery, people must separate themselves from those whom they have depended on for interactions and support. Limited means, burned bridges, and impoverished support all become risk factors for relapse as an individual in recovery struggles to find ways to establish broader circles of healthy social connections. Healthy recovery eventually must include reintegration into broader society.

Roxanna: I was raised to consider community volunteerism to be an essential element of life. A feeling of being valued and accepted comes naturally from participation in neighborhood activities where the goals of meeting social needs are explicit. From the youngest of ages, our family members were introduced to opportunities, programs, and diverse situations that brought a sense of satisfaction in a rapid and rewarding manner. To this day, I clean trash off street corners and perform other unwitnessed acts of service because it is so central to what I have learned is healthy. Some of the group members embraced the philosophy of doing what one can to help those around them, while others seemed to become mired in their own needs.

In the context of the activities that we present in this section, the pleasure of helping others was present. Wisdom comes from diverse sources.

I am reminded of a most rewarding case of transformation with one young woman who sat at a table separated from the larger group. She self-isolated in her posture, her positioning, and her responses to others. While the group attended to the activity, "Advice for the Young," she constructed an elaborate origami wheel. While that was not part of the activity at hand, it turned out that her hobby, prior to becoming addicted to drugs, had been origami. The wheel was constructed with movable spokes that could open and close small windows. In the windows, she wrote words of advice that she "should have" received at various stages of her life. Six spokes identified the ages she would have benefited from the wisdom contained within, and on the corresponding spoke she identified the dates of those missed opportunities. This woman was so gratified with the wheel that she shared her art in the discussion session following the activity. Not revealing the actual advice, she demonstrated the moving parts of the structure and even gave details of the ages she perceived that she could have benefited from the advice. The group was so taken with her creativity and ability, and some began to approach her for words of wisdom. Her interactions with individual group members changed dramatically. By the next week, entirely different social interactions surrounded her, and she requested the opportunity to teach some of her folding skills so that others could construct a simple origami project.

Kay: In active addiction, support circles shrink. Successful recovery involves broadening social support to include not only those in the immediate recovery community but also those in the world at large. Trying new hobbies, volunteering, or doing group service work takes people out of themselves and can increase a sense of belonging. "Free Things to Do" was developed to educate people about the wealth of enrichment opportunities available in the community.

"Curandero Books," "Mandalas," and "Meditation Beads" present activities and concepts that are not part of our typical American traditions but are a part of a world heritage. It is our hope these approaches will increase cultural awarness and give clients a richer base from which to draw inspiration.

"Percussion Band" and "Pass the Wave" are wonderfully spontaneous and uninhibited activities that take on a life of their own and reflect the moods and needs of individual group members.

During the time I worked at the inpatient treatment center, we had an organic garden where clients volunteered their time. Although an entire garden venture is beyond the scope of this book, the experience is worth noting. It proved to be a very therapeutic activity that fostered a strong sense of fellowship. Working together, the residents prepared the raised beds, planted seeds, watered, and weeded. Lettuce, tomatoes, radishes, herbs, and cutting flowers were proudly harvested for the cafeteria. Even those who had no gardening experience enjoyed working in the dirt and contributing to a team project that would benefit the whole treatment community.

"Participants discover that they often share the same uncertainties then are strengthened by the common bond."

Roxanna Erickson-Klein

Advice for the Young

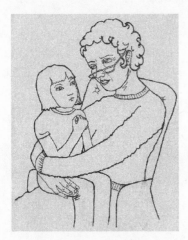

Objectives

- To encourage the process of introspection and thinking through consequences of actions.

- To reinforce the concept that wisdom can be found within oneself and that it is never too late to access that wisdom.

Directions

1. Read the following instructions to the participants:

This is an activity that is personal, but it is also a way to give to others.

This activity helps you remember the time when a strong message MIGHT have helped you. By hearing that message today and sharing it with others, it can help you maintain your recovery.

- *Now think back to the age when you first became aware that using substances was a problem for you.*

- *Now think back to the time when you were unaware, maybe using alcohol or other drugs, but you did not yet know that it was a problem.*

- *And now, think further to the time BEFORE you used and were innocent of how alcohol or other drugs could hurt you.*

- *Ask yourself, "Which time of my life would have been best if SOMEONE had tried to help?"*

- *What words MIGHT have helped you? It is possible that the words were spoken to you but did not sink in. It is possible that those around you were also lost and unable help you. Use the time NOW to hear the words, real or imagined, in your own voice.*

- *Bring your wisdom of TODAY, earned through the hardships you have faced, and write those words.*

Location: Indoors

Time: 60 minutes

Materials: Colored paper

Variety of pens and pencils

Optional: Decorative supplies

- *Send a message to yourself so that you can offer it to the soft and vulnerable parts that are still within you.*

- *Write out the message in pictures or images.*

- *Afterward there will be voluntary sharing with the group.*

2. Ask the group if anyone would like to share their experience.

Observations

This voluntary activity was offered to a group of forty. Instructions were given to use shapes or colors if words could not be found to express ideas. Surprisingly, of such a large group, all participated with the artistic expression; only about ten used words, and the remainder used images. Two participants constructed boxes: one put her resources of comfort within her box, and the other put her anger in her box. One participant designed an elaborate wheel that illustrated various times of her life and what might have helped her during those phases. One constructed a heart and shared with the group that she "just didn't get enough love." About one-third of the participants shared their words/images with the group. The entire group expressed appreciation for the opportunity to participate.

Inspired by: Wisdom passed down by the elders, and Milton Erickson's technique of seeking resources within.

Curandero Books

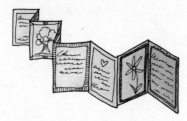

Location: Indoors

Time: 90 minutes

Materials: Legal-size paper

Construction paper

Pens, markers, or colored pencils

Magazines to cut up for illustrations

Rulers

Scissors

Glue

Curandero Books Handout (one per person)

Optional: Scrapbook paper

Objectives

- To focus on emotional healing and the positive power of written words.
- To encourage a creative method of personalizing coping skills.
- To share coping skills with peers.
- To use traditional Mexican folk art as a cultural inspiration.

Directions

1. Prior to the start of the activity, prefold the legal-size paper and construction paper into four panels. Two pieces of the legal-size paper will be glued together to form an eight-panel book, and you might want to glue together the pages ahead of time. If you cut the paper lengthwise participants can make a shorter book.

2. Give each participant the Curandero Book Handout and have a brief discussion about this folk art tradition. This activity is loosely based on a native Mexican healing custom. Additional information can be found online if you wish to expand on this tradition.

3. Review the directions for putting the little books together and encourage participants to decorate them as a personal expression.

4. At the end, ask participants to share with others in small groups.

Observations

Almost all participants were focused and engaged. The finished books were creative and helped demonstrate personal strengths that could be shared with others.

Inspired by: Reading about and seeing photographs of handmade books from Puebla, Mexico.

Curandero Books HANDOUT

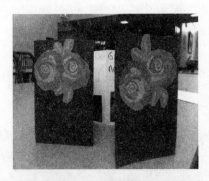

Curanderos are traditional Mexican folk healers. In the village of San Pablito, near Pueblo, Mexico, the curanderos create beautiful hand-decorated books. The books are made from "Papel Amate," which is paper made from tree bark, and have been handcrafted for centuries. These books are typical of the Otomi Indians of this region and are decorated with colorful images that are painted or made from paper cutouts.

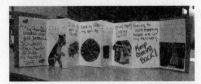

The project we are going to do today uses the curandero books as inspiration. We will make books with a cover and eight pages. Inside each page of the book, you will write one sentence about what makes you feel better when you are sad, what heals your spirits, or something that helps you in your recovery. You can decorate each page using colored paper to make your own designs or pictures from magazines.

DIRECTIONS

1. Choose a piece of colored paper for the front and back covers of your book. These have already been cut to the correct size.

2. Take two pieces of long, white paper for the inside of your book. These have already been cut to the correct size.

3. Glue together two pieces of long white paper so you have eight "pages."

4. Glue the colored paper on the front and on the back.

5. Now write one sentence on each page of your book about something that makes you feel better when you are sad, something that lifts your spirits, or something that helps you in your recovery.

6. Decorate each page with a design you have cut from colored paper or from the pages of a magazine. Decorate the cover of the book. Be creative!

Free Things to Do

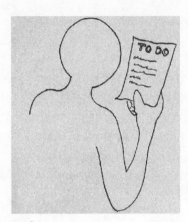

Location: Indoors or Outdoors

Time: 45 minutes

Materials: Copies of advertisements for places around town that offer no cost or low-cost healthy activities

Copies of neighborhood newspapers or local guides to weekly events

Objectives

- To find solutions to the "boredom" that is often cited as a relapse trigger.
- To encourage people to replace unhealthy activities with ones that are positive and pleasurable.

Directions

1. Find and create a list of no-cost or low-cost activities in your community. Refer to ideas on the next page. Suggestions include researching a city's tourism website. Local newspaper activities' guides, sometimes divided by neighborhoods, are good resources. You can also search by activity: art shows, festivals, yoga classes, meditation groups, exercise classes, concerts, performing arts, children's activities, or support groups.

2. Direct participants to sit in a circle.

3. Go around the circle and let each person share something enjoyable they have done in the community in the past that was free or cost very little.

4. Pass out the list and/or newspapers prepared.

5. Ask each person to find something he or she would like to do.

6. Have participants share their choices with the group.

Observations

We found that several people had never participated in any free community events and did not realize they were available. Understanding the options available gave many the initiative to use the suggestions once they left the treatment center and had the freedom to make their own schedule.

Inspired by: The need for people to replace negative behaviors with sober fun.

Suggestions for Finding Free Events in Your Community

- Look in local guides and neighborhood newspapers.
- Go to your city's tourism website or the convention and visitor's bureau.
- Search online for meetup groups in your area.

Arts and culture: Find shows or exhibitions at museums, galleries, outdoor art shows, and art walks.

History: Often there are free festivals or displays in historic areas.

Outdoors: Depending on your geographic location, look for parks, recreation areas, wilderness trails, exercise trails, and farmers' markets.

Music: Symphonies and orchestras often sponsor free concerts, sometimes outdoors or in churches. Look for youth orchestras, groups from neighboring communities, drum circles, and dance groups.

Libraries: Often they sponsor free events and celebrations for families and children or free classes.

Exercise: City parks, museums, dance studios, and yoga studios offer free exercise classes. Biking clubs, running clubs, and sports stores have events aimed at all fitness levels and ages. Many community centers, local gyms, or even sports stores have training classes, boot camps, and sample classes. Exercise studios sometimes offer free or low cost classes one day per week.

Educate: Historical societies, museums, community colleges, and universities sponsor talks and brown bag lunch lectures.

Give back: Many volunteer opportunities are available through local charities or nonprofits. Look up charity walks or projects that help you get exercise, meet others, and give back to the community at the same time. Check out Random Acts of Kindness, Habitat for Humanity, animal shelters, domestic violence shelters, children's groups, and elder support.

Spiritual: Churches, synagogues, mosques, and temples host free events. Also look at meditation centers.

Support: Local mental health organizations, nonprofits, hospitals, and churches sponsor various support groups. A variety of twelve-step groups are found in almost every town.

Group Thoughts on Recovery

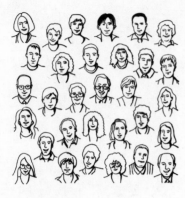

Location: Indoors

Time: 45–90 minutes (depending on size of group)

Materials: Pens or pencils

Group Thoughts on Recovery Handout (one per group)

Objectives

- To explore the realities of sobriety in a positive way.

- To work as a group with a common interest in recovery.

- To encourage the group to think about the concept of recovery in relation to the ideas of friendship, curiosity, leadership, intelligence, good luck, happiness, and hope.

Directions

1. Prior to the activity, cut the Group Thoughts on Recovery Handout into seven sections as marked.

2. Divide the group into seven groups.

3. Ask each group to select one person as the writer or note taker. Another person should be selected to be the reporter who will share a summary with the larger group at the end.

4. Give each group one set of questions from the handout to fill out and discuss.

5. Allow about twenty minutes for group discussions.

6. When individual groups are finished, reconvene the whole group to discuss their thoughts and insights.

Observations

This activity was done is a large group of forty participants. Sometimes participants who have relapsed blame circumstances, such as "My boyfriend left me" or "My mother died." This helped them realize that recovery is not contingent on external factors. Participants were not advised in advance that each series of questions are identical, with different topics. As the groups discovered this, the discussion became very animated and dynamic. Overall, the variations in perspective were interesting and insightful. At the conclusion, the group elected to construct a larger list of factors believed to influence recovery. The group-generated list included honesty, self-respect, courage, strength, discipline, guilt, maturity, and freedom.

Inspired by: The success of peers in broadening an individual's optimism about recovery.

Group Thoughts on Recovery HANDOUT

Give each group the section with its topic.

Questions on Friendship

1. What does friendship have to do with recovery?

2. Is friendship a good thing or a bad thing?

3. Does friendship lead you toward recovery or away from it?

4. Can friendship get you into trouble in recovery?

5. How would you know if friendship is helping or hurting you?

6. Do you have any thoughts about friendship that you want to share with the group?

Questions on Curiosity

1. What does curiosity have to do with recovery?

2. Is curiosity a good thing or a bad thing?

3. Does curiosity lead you toward recovery or away from it?

4. Can curiosity get you into trouble in recovery?

5. How would you know if curiosity is helping or hurting you?

6. Do you have any thoughts about curiosity that you want to share with the group?

Questions on Leadership

1. What does leadership have to do with recovery?

2. Is leadership a good thing or a bad thing?

3. Does leadership lead you toward recovery or away from it?

4. Can leadership get you into trouble in recovery?

5. How would you know if leadership is helping or hurting you?

6. Do you have any thoughts about leadership that you want to share with the group?

Questions on Intelligence

1. What does intelligence have to do with recovery?

2. Is intelligence a good thing or a bad thing?

3. Does intelligence lead you toward recovery or away from it?

4. Can intelligence get you into trouble in recovery?

5. How would you know if intelligence is helping or hurting you?

6. Do you have any thoughts about intelligence that you want to share with the group?

Questions on Good Luck

1. What does good luck have to do with recovery?

2. Is good luck a good thing or a bad thing?

3. Does good luck lead you toward recovery or away from it?

4. Can good luck get you into trouble in recovery?

5. How would you know if good luck is helping or hurting you?

6. Do you have any thoughts about good luck that you want to share with the group?

Questions on Happiness

1. What does happiness have to do with recovery?

2. Is happiness a good thing or a bad thing?

3. Does happiness lead you toward recovery or away from it?

4. Can happiness get you into trouble in recovery?

5. How would you know if happiness is helping or hurting you?

6. Do you have any thoughts about happiness that you want to share with the group?

Questions on Hope

1. What does hope have to do with recovery?

2. Is hope a good thing or a bad thing?

3. Does hope lead you toward recovery or away from it?

4. Can hope get you into trouble in recovery?

5. How would you know if hope is helping or hurting you?

6. Do you have any thoughts about hope that you want to share with the group?

Human Tic-Tac-Toe

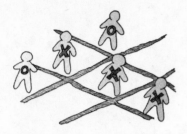

Location: Outdoors or Indoors

Time: 20 minutes

Materials: Chalk on cement, ribbons, or pieces of rope

6 Xs and 6 Os (copy from illustrations provided)

Token prizes

Human Tic-Tac-Toe Handout (one per person)

Objectives

- To foster a friendly atmosphere inclusive of serious discussion about recovery.

- To recognize that others may answer serious questions in different ways.

- To provide an opportunity for individuals to make critical judgments while in a safe group setting.

Directions

1. Draw a large tic-tac-toe grid with chalk or place ribbons or rope to make a grid on the ground large enough for people to stand in or sit in.

2. Divide participants into X and O teams.

3. Present participants with a copy of the Human Tic-Tac-Toe Handout.

4. Instruct teams to huddle and decide which question to answer. Tell participants that the answer must be longer than a short phrase, and the group must reach a consensus on the answer to the question.

5. Team X begins. Ask the first player to announce the question and explain the answer the team agreed upon. Then instruct the team to place a team member on the grid.

6. Next ask a representative from Team O to to read aloud a question, present the team's answer, and then take a position on the grid. Each team can use a question only once. There are no "right" answers; any thoughtful response is acceptable.

7. Award winning team members with small prizes.

Observations

This game was played in an outdoor setting with thirty women in recovery and again played in a smaller group with students with various disabilities in an indoor setting. Questions were modified for the latter group. In each case, the questions stimulated lively discussion regarding the values underlying the topics. Teams went back to questions they felt the opposite team had not properly addressed. With the student group, this game was played for more than an hour, but with the recovery group the game was used in combination with other outdoor activities and lasted about twenty minutes.

Inspired by: Adapted from outdoor games for children.

Human Tic-Tac-Toe HANDOUT

When do you know that you are safe in recovery?

How do you handle cravings?

How can you help someone else in recovery ?

What can you do to prevent or discourage kids from using substances?

Why not enjoy another substance that is different from your drug of choice?

How long does it take before someone recognizes he or she is addicted?

What advice would you give to children to prevent use of alcohol or other drugs?

How can you show your sponsor how much you appreciate him or her?

How will you handle it if you are at a party and everyone else has wine or a beer?

How can you approach someone you respect when you suspect he or she may be abusing substances?

Is it morally wrong to abuse alcohol or other drugs?

Is it important to listen to each of the instructional class sessions even if you have heard it before?

What makes the difference from knowing what you need to do in recovery and actually doing it?

Can you help someone who is not yet ready to be helped?

What is the use of going through the recovery process if you might relapse later?

Can you be proud of yourself even if you have made bad choices?

What's the problem with taking a hit of something after you have completely recovered?

What is the hardest part of recovery?

Is being in treatment supposed to be fun?

What will you remember most about this time in your life?

Is being at a recovery center supposed to be fun?

What will you remember most about this stage in your recovery?

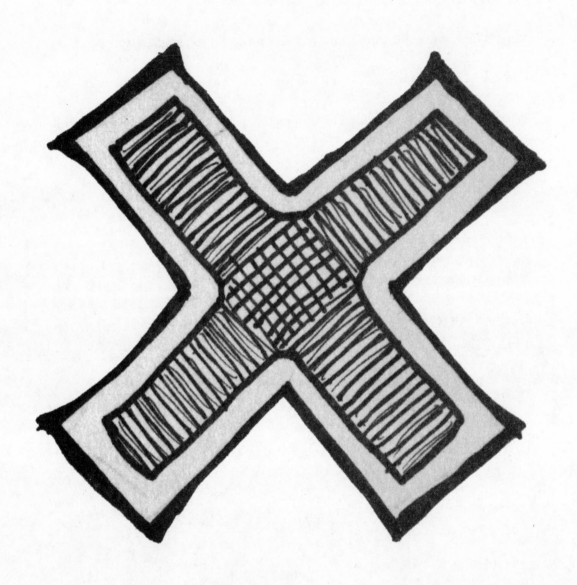

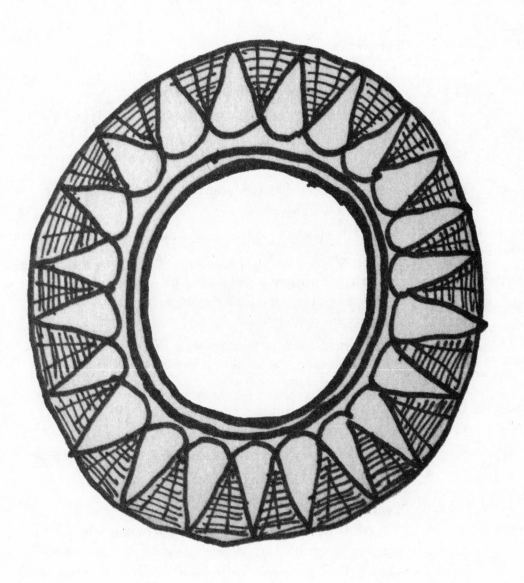

Mandalas

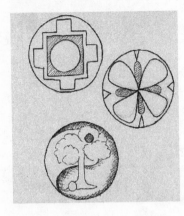

Location: Indoors

Time: 30–45 minutes

Materials: Plain drawing paper

Pens, markers, or colored pencils

A circle to trace (can be a coffee can lid or similar size)

Mandalas Handout (one per person)

Optional: Soothing music to play

Objectives

- To demonstrate mindfulness skills.
- To help participants focus and find meaning.
- To engage in a cross-cultural method of envisioning one's place in the universe.

Directions

1. Conduct a brief discussion with the group about mandalas using the Mandala Handout.

2. Provide examples of various designs from books or from online resources.

3. Instruct participants to gather at a table to create an original mandala pattern but explain they are not to speak to each other as they are working. This is a period of silent work.

4. Tell participants to set an intention or have something in mind to focus on as they draw, such as their recovery or meaningful things in their life.

5. Play soothing meditation music or soft jazz music in the background, if possible.

6. Encourage participants to share the story behind their original mandala drawings.

Observations

This activity started as a way to use time creatively after a stress-reduction group. It was extremely popular and was instantly engaging. Playing calming music during the drawing activity and asking participants not to speak enhanced the meditative atmosphere. Many requested mandala "coloring sheets" to use outside of class. Online sites have mandala templates for coloring in. It is strongly recommended that group members be encouraged to create their own patterns first. Once these are completed, other mandalas may be distributed. The participants finished mandalas represented family, recovery, and favorite images.

Inspired by: Numerous cultural traditions that use circular artwork, wheels, and mandalas in healing.

Mandalas HANDOUT

A mandala is a geometric design that symbolizes the world that is within us as well as the world beyond us. The term *mandala* is a Sanskrit word that means "disk" or "circle." Each design begins with a center point and extends from that point. When complete it represents wholeness.

Seen in various spiritual traditions, mandalas can focus a person's attention and be a teaching tool for establishing a sacred space. Also they can be used as an aid to meditation.

Mandalas can be seen throughout the world.

- Indians in the Americas create medicine wheels and sand mandalas.

- The yin-yang symbol, which originated in Asia, is a mandala.

- Mandalas in Tibet often have detailed illustrations with religious meaning and are used for meditation.

- The Navajo, as well as Tibetan monks, create sand mandalas to demonstrate that life is not permanent.

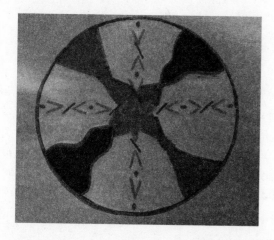

By using different colors, symbols, and patterns that are meaningful to you, a mandala drawing can represent the whole universe in a circle or YOUR universe. It can help you center yourself and get in touch with your own inner reality.

If you made your own personal mandala, what colors would you choose? What is important to you in life? What things might you include in your circle?

Meditation Beads

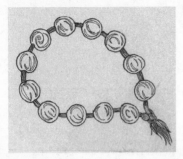

Location: Indoors

Time: 60 minutes

Materials: Variety of beads (about 30 or more for long necklaces, about 10 for bracelets)

Stringing materials

Scissors

Meditation Beads Handout (one per person)

Glue (to reinforce knots on most materials)

Optional: Clasps

Objectives

- To provide novelty and enrichment that engages a variety of ways for decision making and problem solving.

Directions

1. Make one or two samples for the group to see.

2. Read aloud the overview of cultural traditions that have persisted over the millennia that show how people find comfort and spirituality associated with holding, feeling, and manipulating beads.

   The Catholic rosary, Buddhist prayer beads, Armenian worry beads, and even Grandma's pearl necklace provide tangible reminders that beads have an intrinsic way of helping someone who is seeking to find internal calm or strengthen faith. Each of these different traditions has its own meaningful number of beads.

   - *Buddhists and Hindu malas have 18, 21, 27, or 108.*
   - *Catholic rosaries have 108.*
   - *Muslim tesbih have 33 or 99.*
   - *Greek komboloi have 33.*
   - *Armenian worry beads have 17 or 33.*

   These strings of beads may be used in various ways: meditation, prayer, to increase faith, hope, and charity, or for saying a personal mantra. Counting the beads can be used as a diversion to break a bad habit. They can contain symbols of our beliefs, good luck, or representations of our strengths and our personality. The act of focusing on the feel or the movement of the worry beads can relax the mind.

3. Ask participants to think about constructing a personal set of meditation beads that reflect their recovery.

4. Show samples of simply constructed strings of beads, along with instructions on how to tie a square knot on the Meditation Beads Handout.

5. Invite participants to select their own beads, string, and design.

6. Allow about thirty minutes for selection and stringing.

7. Invite participants to show what they have constructed and how it will help them in recovery.

Observations

This activity was done three times with two different groups of ten and again with a larger group of thirty. Each time the participants spent a lot of time thinking about what would be most meaningful to them. The creations were varied, and there were certain materials that were highly prized, including alphabet beads and stretch string. With the stretch string it is very important to tie the knot extremely tight so that it does not unwind. The number of meditation beads used by participants varied. As the participants worked, adaptation and compromises were needed, as they couldn't find a specific color or size of bead that was desired. Outcomes included twelve beads for the Twelve Steps, the number of days of recovery, number of children or family members, and the number of days she had spent incarcerated. Carefully chosen beads reflected colors and designs to correspond with the meaning behind them. Some participants selected strings to hold the beads securely in position, and other designs allowed for some movement of the bead along the string. In each case, the symbolic representations were personal, meaningful, and soothing in their own way. The experience provided a diversion with tangible outcomes that enhanced ongoing interpersonal communication.

Inspired by: An appreciation for diverse multicultural uses of beads.

Meditation Beads HANDOUT

How to Tie a Square Knot
(optional)

A square knot starts just like tying a bow, but the next step repeats the first, going in the opposite direction. A simple way to remember how to tie a square knot is to say, "Right over left, left over right."

To begin: Use either two pieces or one long piece of rope, string, or ribbon. If you use a single piece, it may be helpful to mark one of the ends so that you can identify one from the other. This diagram refers to the two ends as the light rope and the dark rope.

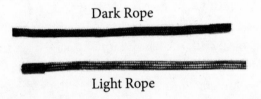

Dark Rope

Light Rope

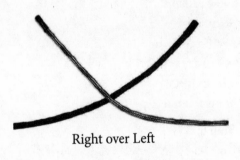

Right over Left

Step 1: Lay down each rope horizontally as shown above.

Step 2: Drape the light rope over the dark rope and form a large X. Right over left.

Step 3: Tuck the light rope under the dark rope.

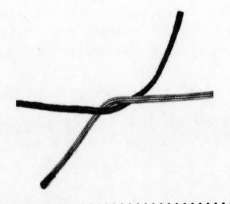

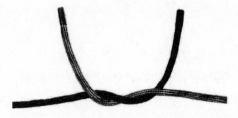

Step 4: Bring the end of the light rope back over the dark rope to form a loose single knot.

Step 5: Form another X with the two ends, making sure the light rope is on top of the dark one. Left over right.

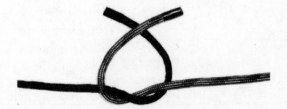

Left over Right

Step 6: Wrap the light end around the dark rope and pull it through the loop.

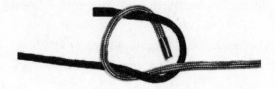

Step 7: Pull the two ends tightly to finish the knot. You're done!

My Life Network

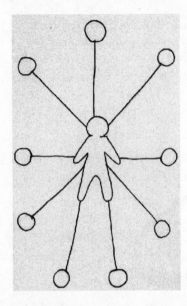

Location: Indoors

Time: 45 minutes

Materials: Pens

Blank paper

Colored pencils

Objectives

- To provide an opportunity to inventory one's own life, including demands and responsibilities.

- To offer a way to objectively observe the relative proportions of strengths and demands.

- To help individuals evaluate strengths and weaknesses in their support system.

Directions

1. Demonstrate using your own life network or ask a volunteer to draw on the board so the participants will see the intuitive pattern.

2. Make a circle in the center of the paper with your name and today's date, about the size of a silver dollar.

3. Construct a few spokes out from the center circle, and make additional circles on those spokes.

4. In the new circles, write recovery, housing, family, finances, health concerns, and any other aspect of life that is important at this time. Participants choose what and how many to include.

5. From each of the smaller circles, draw smaller spokes leading to other circles. And in the circles, identify elements that are important. For example, the recovery circle would have attached circles for sponsor, twelve-step group, outpatient programs, and cravings.

6. For each of the circles surrounding the self, identify elements that are related, yet independent for each of the circles.

7. Once the major aspects of current life are drawn out, use colored pencils to identify which are positive and which are negative.

8. Look over the whole picture and notice whether the majority of the energy is positive or negative.

Observations

This activity was done numerous times in a variety of group settings. Few participants had any difficulty in grasping the concept, and all of them were able to compartmentalize thinking to isolate different life concerns. There was significant ambivalence in identifying positive versus negative energy flow, and several participants came up with creative ways to illustrate that. A few were surprised to see that their networks were weighted heavily on the negative side. Several participants volunteered to share their network with the group for discussion. This activity is a simple and effective tool for individuals to have visual feedback about their lives and to take a personal snapshot to revisit at a later point in time.

Inspired by: Ecomaps, genograms, and social support mapping, which are a staple of social work and family systems work. This is a simple variation of an activity designed by Gary John, EdD.

Example of a Network Recovery Section

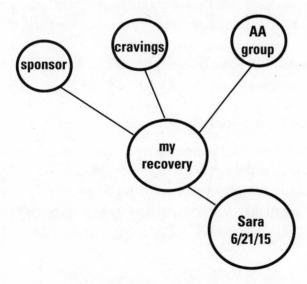

Pass the Wave

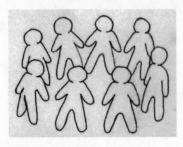

Location: Indoors or Outdoors

Time: 20–45 minutes

Materials: None

Objectives

- To increase focus and attention and practice taking turns and following directions.

- To have people both physically and mentally engaged in a group activity.

Directions

1. Instruct participants to form a large circle.

2. Depending on time constraints, there are several alternate sequences that can be done. Choose one or more of the sequences below.

Pass the Motion Around Circle: The facilitator does a series of movements that will be "passed" around the circle from right to left. The key here is for people to wait and *watch the person next to them*, not to follow the facilitator. Movements can be anything, but here are suggestions: stomp feet, hands smacking thighs, snapping fingers, rubbing palms together, clapping, or hands in the air.

Individual Introduction, Group Reply: Each person says his or her name and comes up with a statement about him- or herself and an action. The first person takes a step into the circle and says his or her name, statement, and performs the action. Example: "My name is Mary, and I like to play baseball." Mary then makes a motion like she is throwing a baseball. Then the rest of the circle in *unison* will repeat the person's name, statement, and perform the action.

Group Wave: First person starts a motion (hands raised up, for example) and the person next to them picks up the motion, while the first person also continues. A "wave" of motion forms as the action goes around the circle to include everyone.

Pass the Motion in a Random Style: First person will pass a motion (hand clap, finger snap, or other gesture) toward another person, who will then pass on the gesture to a third person, and so on. People choose each other by eye contact, by a head movement, or by calling a name. They do not have to choose the person next to them—the motion can jump across the circle. Only the selected person does the movement.

3. Explain the rules of the first sequence you select.

4. Have the movement continue until it goes the whole way around the circle and back to the beginning, so everyone has a turn.

Observations

People in the very early stages of recovery often have memory and cognitive functioning challenges. This was an excellent activity to help stimulate focusing and following a pattern. In the first activity, there were many times people did the movement too soon because they were not watching their neighbor carefully. We have noticed a hyper-alert awareness in some participants that interferes with healthy social interaction. In the discussion period, some participants revealed feeling uncomfortable having others watch them. This activity provides a nonthreatening way to be an active member of a group.

As the activity progressed, even those reluctant to join in were actively engaged by the time the second round started. Some used small gestures such as a thumbs up. Others performed elaborate dance moves. The group laughed a lot and many commented that they had a great time, and this was just what they needed to lift their mood.

Inspired by: Various team building group activities done at workshops and crowd waves at sporting events.

Percussion Band

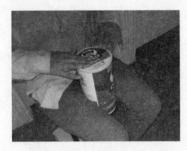

Objectives

- To provide a means of expression through sound.
- To engage in a cooperative exploratory expression of one's feelings.
- To promote play, release anger, encourage teamwork, and build a sense of community.

Directions

1. Arrange chairs in a circle in an area where noise will not be problematic for adjacent work areas. Participants can also sit in a circle outside on the grass.

2. Ask each participant to select an instrument.

3. Instruct everyone to sit in a circle with you in the center. Create a gesture that will communicate to the group when to start and when to stop playing.

4. **Round A: All Join In**

   A. First person begins with a slow steady beat of his or her choosing and continues this throughout the round.

   B. Next person starts with his or her own, complementary beat and continues to play.

   C. Third person joins in with his or her beat and continues to play.

   D. Continue until the entire circle is playing.

   E. When full circle is engaged, gesture for a crescendo.

   F. Conclude with all instruments stopping simultaneously.

7. **Round B: A Moving Wave of Sound**

   A. One person begins with a simple, distinct pattern of a beat. For example, TAH—TAH—TAH-TAH-TAH (repeat)

   B. The first player stops. A second person imitates the same beat.

   C. Continue around the circle with each member playing individually.

Location: Indoors or Outdoors

Time: 60 minutes

Materials: Homemade or actual percussion instruments (one for each participant)

Household items to make instruments (shoeboxes; cookie tins; small boxes with beans or paper clips; buckets; wooden sticks to bang on a box or to bang together; empty paper towel tubes filled with beans, rice, or pasta and sealed with duct tape)

Whiteboard

Markers

4. **Round C: Putting a Beat to Words**

    A. Ask a volunteer for a word, short poem, rap, or phrase that is meaningful to his or her personal recovery.

    B. Write the word or phrase on a whiteboard.

    C. The same volunteer explains what the phrase would sound like in rhythm.

    D. Note on the whiteboard where the beat or emphasis will be and what instruments are to play and when. The volunteer can help orchestrate this.

    E. The volunteer then repeatedly reads the phrase or speaks the word.

    F. The group follows the instructions, says the phrase, and taps out the sounds as directed.

    G. Have another volunteer offer a word or phrase.

    H. Continue until all volunteers have had an opportunity to have their words expressed musically.

Observations

This activity was performed with a group of thirty participants and two facilitators, who did not have a musical background or musical talent. The preponderance of the instruments were shoe boxes, some tapped by hand and others with chopsticks for drum sticks. Two bass drums (large paint buckets turned upside down) were delegated to participants with strong musical backgrounds who were enthusiastic about keeping the beat. Numerous shakers were constructed from small tins filled with beans or paper clips, and wooden sticks of various diameters were quite useful.

The day of this activity was dreary and rainy. The group attitude prior to the activity was lethargic and withdrawn. As with most of the activities, a few individuals were slow to join, initially sitting back to observe the session. One, fearful of migraine headaches, asked to be excused. After the initial round, the unexpected harmonies produced were successful in engaging all group members in a cheerful, cooperative, and energetic sharing experience. The enthusiasm was palpable. The concept of self-care and healing in para-verbal expression seemed to be both understood and embraced.

The initial design of this activity involved a round with a conductor in the center of the circle, directing participants to play or hush and changing the speed and volume of the tempo. While this may be a useful technique for experienced musicians, it proved to be too challenging for our group.

When we performed the third session, involving words and phrases (Round C), about a third of the participants jumped in, clearly enjoying the leadership role as well as the chance to explore their own meanings. Some of the phrases were clearly related to recovery, while others were song lyrics or personal statements. One phrase offered by a participant was: "I fly like a butterfly, sting like a bee, I am my recovery, my recovery is me."

Inspired by: This activity was originally inspired by an article that appeared in a professional journal by Michael Winkelman, PhD. The activity that appears here is not nearly as structured or refined as was described in the article.

We would also like to thank Sara Brown, LCDC, at Nexus for her helpful suggestions.

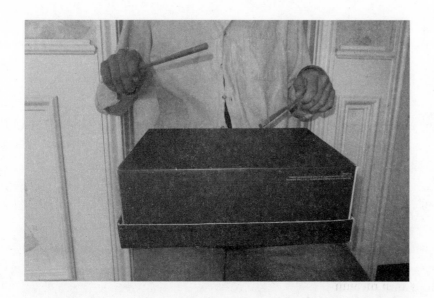

Creative use of ordinary household items for percussion instruments.

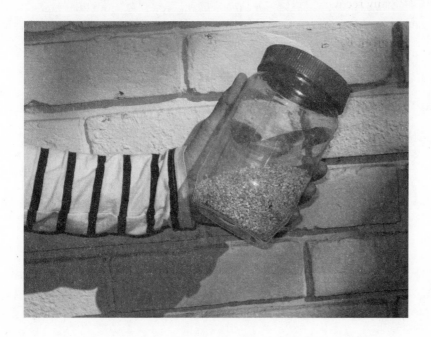

Recovery Quilt

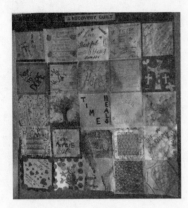

Location: Indoors

Time: 90–120 minutes

Materials: Construction paper or scrapbook paper (cut into 8½-inch squares)

Colored pens, markers, or paint, fabric paint

Glitter, sequins, or collage materials

Duct tape

Curtain rod, shower rod, or wooden dowel

Recovery Quilt Handout (one per person)

Objectives

- To have clients create an image that tells something about their personal journey.
- To have clients come together to create a larger picture of recovery.
- To reflect on quilting tradition in America.

Directions

1. Using the Recovery Quilt Handout, have a short discussion with the group about the cultural history of quilting and how it has been used to tell stories in the past for those who were not part of mainstream society. Ask if anyone has any relative who likes to make quilts.

2. Have each participant create a personal square with words, pictures, or collage.

3. Attach each completed square to the other by using duct tape along the back. Start with top row and continue to add squares.

4. Hang the assembled quilt from a rod in a public area.

Observations

Participants enjoyed contributing to this quilt and were proud of the finished product. This activity was done once in recognition of Black History Month in February. Another time, it was done in celebration of an anniversary of the treatment facility. Participants engaged cooperatively to make unique designs. Most wanted to share their work with the group. The finished quilt was hung on a wall, which allowed participants to stand in front and show their squares.

Inspired by: The tradition of quilting and observation of Black History Month.

Recovery Quilt HANDOUT

Harriet Powers was born into slavery in Georgia in 1837. She made quilts which are the best known examples of the Southern American quilting tradition. Using traditional appliqué techniques, Harriet recorded local legends, Bible stories, and astronomical occurrences in her quilts.

Quilt Facts

Quilts are a collection of images that tell a story.

The stories can represent:

- Love
- Events
- Friendship
- Teamwork
- History
- Beauty
- Scarce resources
- Traditions

The quilts themselves become a story. They tell:

- The work and how much time they had.
- Attention to detail.
- Who did it ? One person or a group?
- Why?
- What materials were available?

Our Recovery Quilt

The purpose of this quilt is to bring together thoughts about yourself in recovery.

What theme do you want for the quilt?

Can we come together as a team . . .

- in a short time?
- with not too many materials?
- and create an image of recovery?

What will the quilt look like?

What will it be like to be part of the process?

Snowflakes

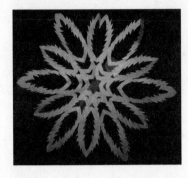

Location: Indoors

Time: 60 minutes

Materials: Tissue paper in white or various colors

Scratch paper

Scissors

Scotch tape

Individual trash receptacles (paper plates work well)

Objectives

- To reflect upon the unique and changing beauty in nature and appreciate the unique beauty of individuals.

- To create a decorative, seasonal atmosphere in which holidays are appreciated.

Directions

1. Prior to the activity, search for a poem about snowflakes and display the poem for everyone to see. Begin the activity by reading the poem aloud.

2. Pass out scratch paper, scissors, and individual trash receptacles.

3. Begin with a large, square piece of paper.

   A. Fold in half diagonally to make a triangle shape.

   B. Fold again, to make a triangle that is now one-fourth the size of the original square.

   C. Fold one-third of the way over. At this time, some points will stick out further than others.

   D. Fold again so that the thirds are all stacked, with points sticking out irregularly from the open end. It may be necessary to adjust the first third fold as it is hard to estimate.

   E. Cut off the ends that stick out. After cutting it will look like a smooth triangle again.

   F. Cut shapes from each side of the triangle.

   G. Unfold.

4. Distribute large tissue paper sheets for participants to create snowflakes.

5. Tape the tissue snowflakes to walls or windows for a beautiful collage.

6. Invite participants to comment about the process.

Observations

The snowflake activity was done in early December using large sheets of colored tissue paper and remained during the holidays for translucent window decor. For lower-functioning group members, there is an alternate way to fold using only halves and avoiding the one-third fold. It produces an eight-sided snowflake which is also beautiful. The participants in this group compiled the following list of comments about the activity:

- Beauty is all around us.

- Nothing is perfect.

- When the imperfections are accepted, a new type of beauty shows itself.

- Nothing ever comes out exactly the way we plan it.

- With practice, we are better able to control the outcome.

- No matter how hard you try, there is something to clean up afterward.

- Clean up your own mess.

- Learn from others, and then create our own images.

- Exploring new skills can be safe and fun.

- It does not take a lot of material things to bring happiness.

- There are a lot of pleasant ways to relax.

Inspired by: A poem titled "Each of Us a Snowflake," attributed to Emily Warburton.

Spirit Sticks

Location: Indoors

Time: 90 minutes

Materials: 1 stick or wooden dowel per person (approximately 12 inches in length)

String, yarn, ribbon, or thin wire

yarn, material remnants, or decorative paper

assortment of small objects for stringing (beads, buttons, seashells, acorns, or feathers)

glue, tape, or duct tape

markers

scissors

Spirit Sticks Handout (one per person)

Objectives

- To facilitate creation of something symbolic that represents strengths and is meaningful in recovery.

- To engage in a therapeutic project that uses nonverbal expression as a means of communication.

- To raise awareness of multicultural resources that can augment recovery.

Directions

1. Begin a short discussion with the group about the origin of spirit sticks in Native American culture, using the Spirit Sticks Handout.

2. Encourage participants to create something that has meaning for them in their life and in their recovery, choosing items that represent inner strengths, skills, or special people in their lives.

3. If feasible, allow participants to collect items from outdoors to use, such as leaves, acorns, feathers, or small rocks.

4. Arrange materials on a table and have everyone work on their personal sticks.

5. When all participants have finished, invite volunteers to explain to the group the meaning of the items on their personal spirit stick.

Observations

This activity engaged everyone in the group and took the entire ninety minutes. Participants displayed creativity and originality in the creation of their spirit sticks. Almost all participants wanted to share their finished project with the group. Many demonstrated good reflection and the ability to recognize and symbolize touchstones or precious elements in their lives.

Inspired by: A former client who made spirit sticks as gifts for others.

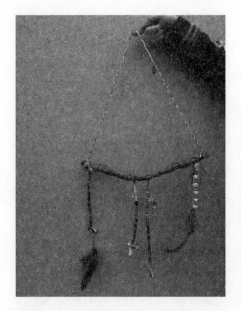

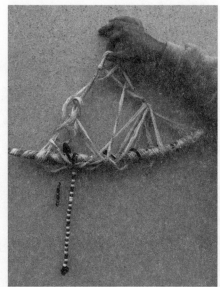

Different colored beads and objects represent long-term, family, and goals in life.

Elaborate webbing on this stick symbolized complicated life patterns.

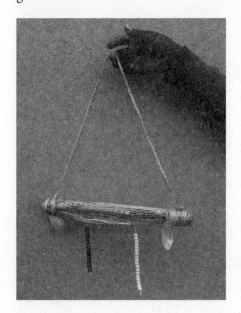

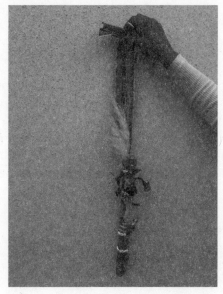

A representation of past anger and future, positive energy.

A photo of a child was incorporated into this design.

Spirit Sticks HANDOUT

Some Native American shamans, or medicine men and women, use special decorated sticks called spirit sticks. These are usually sticks decorated with items from nature, such as feathers, pieces of animal fur, animal teeth, or claws. They may also be decorated with beads, ribbons, or other items. These sticks are used for sacred ceremonies and to help answer prayers.

Today, we are going to use this tradition as inspiration to make our own spirit sticks.

Take a stick and think about decorating it with items that have significance for you in your life and in your recovery. Try to create something that you can use to give you strength and intention. Perhaps the stick will help you in your healing journey, replacing negative thoughts with positive ones. It might represent your inner strengths or skills.

You might write yourself an encouraging slogan or message to attach or draw something or even find something from nature to add.

You might paint your stick or wrap in paper or fabric.

Choose items that have some meaning for you and attach them to your stick with yarn or string.

"We don't yet understand scientifically how actions contribute to healing, but I don't think there is any doubt that getting engaged in creative activities moves the process forward."

Roxanna Erickson-Klein

Twelve-Step Banner

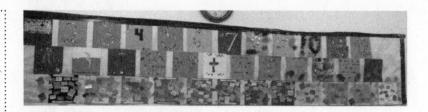

Location: Indoors

Time: Two sequential, 90-minute sessions (can be a week apart and can include some participant turnover)

Materials: Banner paper (long enough for 36 squares, at least 24-feet long)

Tables or workspace (sufficient to display banner and have participants approach and glue own comments about the Twelve Steps)

12" × 12" construction paper squares

Small pastel note cards (1" × 2", in a variety of colors, about 500)

Pens

Glue or glue sticks

Duct tape

Various art supplies

The Twelve Steps (one per person; see Appendix.)

Objectives

- To create a banner for public display.
- To engage in group planning and problem solving.
- To familiarize the participants with the twelve-step methodology.
- To reflect upon personal perspectives of moving through the Twelve Steps.

Directions

SESSION ONE

1. Place precut banner paper on a long table or work area. Put all other supplies on a nearby table.

2. Hand out copies of the Alcoholics Anonymous and Narcotics Anonymous Twelve Steps. Review objectives for the project as a whole. Explain that at the end of the first session, it is expected that two squares will be completed: one with the number of each step and the second with a visual representation of what each step means.

3. Ask volunteers to be team leaders for each step. Participants can choose any step number, regardless of their own progress (one team per step).

4. Ask team leaders select other team members so there are equal numbers of participants on each team.

5. Ask each team leader to choose two 12" × 12" construction paper squares, any color.

6. Instruct each team leader to plan with team members how to design their step number and what sort of a visual representation will be on the second square.

7. Remind teams to use arts and craft materials and turn in their squares at the end of the session.

SESSION TWO

8. Pass out additional handouts of Alcoholics Anonymous and Narcotics Anonymous.

9. Display banner in work area. Ask volunteers to help with the layout of the existing squares and making space for a third set of squares.

   • Position Steps 1–12 on the top row.

   • On the second row, place the visual representations of the corresponding steps.

   • On the third row, place blank squares, awaiting individual comments about each step. The three squares representing each step can be positioned under each other making a straight column, or they can be offset.

10. Instruct a team of volunteers to align and glue the squares in place, while the rest of the group uses note cards to compose personal reflections of each of the Twelve Steps.

11. Once the assembly is complete, invite team leaders and team members to describe their work to the larger group. At the end of each step description, invite members from the larger group to speak about their contribution.

12. Once all the Twelve Steps have been described by the assigned teams and the participants in the larger group have had a chance to comment on their personal reaction, individuals post personal comments or reflections on the bottom row of note cards.

Observations

This activity was conducted with twelve teams with three participants each. Each team took their roles and their autonomy seriously, creating an interesting variety of displays. In the second session, participants embraced the activity with a cooperative spirit. Many remarked they learned more about the Twelve Steps in those two sessions than they had learned before. Universally, it was described as useful to envision oneself at a later point in time facing future steps.

Inspired by: The flexibility of the twelve-step model to draw out peer leadership skills.

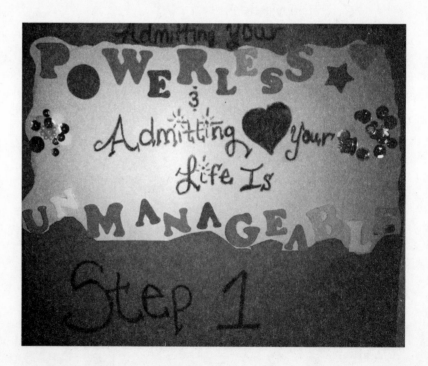

A closeup of Step 1.

"Trust your steps on a
well-established path."

KAY COLBERT

Windows to the World

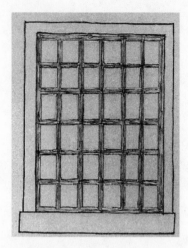

Objectives

- To work as a team.
- To create a mutually agreeable display in recognition of an event.

Directions

1. Prepare the following before the session begins:

   A. Decide on a theme for the banner. We decided to celebrate Earth Day, but any holiday or event can be utilized.

   B. Sketch a rough draft for the finished banner and prepare samples of one window and one shutter to show the group.

   C. Identify a location where the completed banner can be displayed. Prepare one example of a window and a shutter.

   D. Count the number of letters in the name of the celebration or event for the banner. For example, "Earth Day April 22" has 15 letters. Assure the banner paper is sufficiently long enough to accommodate the full message that will be displayed on the 12" × 12" squares.

5. Tell the group that each letter will represent one team. In the Earth Day example, 15 teams and one additional team to lay out and assemble the banner makes a total of 16 teams.

6. Instruct the teams to select two sheets of 12" × 12" construction paper. One sheet is the shutter and one sheet is the window.

7. On the shutter, have teams write the letter to be displayed or glue a cut out letter on it. For example, the teams for "Earth Day" are assigned the letters E, A, R, T, H, D, A, Y.

8. For the window, tell each team to creatively decorate a square of paper to illustrate the theme.

Location: Indoors

Time: 60–90 minutes

Materials: Banner paper (at least 30 inches tall and long enough to display a series of windows)

Construction paper (12" × 12", various colors)

Various art supplies

Duct tape

Glue

Scissors

9. Inform teams that they'll need to figure out how to get both the shutter letter and the window illustration created.

10. Once the shutter with the letter is completed, direct the team to report to the Assembly Team for placement on the banner paper.

11. Explain the installation process to the Assembly Team:

    A. First place the window illustration on the banner.

    B. Then, use duct tape along one edge of the shutter to affix it over the window, creating a hinge to open and display the window underneath. This results in an interactive display that reveals the hidden beauty when opened.

12. On completion of the work, have team members gather to discuss the experience of working together.

Observations

"Windows to the World" was done as an Earth Day activity but is suitable for any periodic celebration. The group that created the Earth Day display was made up of forty-two participants, so some teams had two members and some teams had three members. The Assembly Team had three members with artistic ability. Assembly is the most challenging part of the group project.

Discussion about working with other teams members was positive and served to bring cohesiveness and a sense of belonging. Although some of the displays were more artistic than others, pride in the overall presentation was rewarding for all involved. Variations in style of composing the letters on the shutters did not present any problems, as the context and words pulled it all together. The finished banner was colorful and creative. The ability to open and close the shutters produced an ongoing interactive piece of group art.

Inspired by: Looking at a country home with shutters on the windows.

Envisioning a Future of Recovery: Anticipation of Holidays and Success Over Time

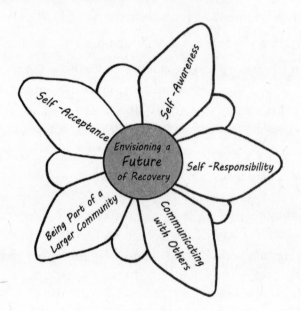

In the addiction field, we say abstinence is not the same as recovery. A period of sobriety may be achieved, but an individual remains at high risk for relapse for a prolonged interval. Inpatient treatment is not the end result but the beginning of a lifelong process. Envisioning a long horizon of freedom from addiction is an important tool that can increase probability of success. This section includes activities specifically targeted to help navigate recovery through difficult times.

Individual crises, whether they are circumstantial, interpersonal, or health related, can stimulate a cascade of events that weaken the probability of success in recovery. "Give Yourself a Checkup" and "Self-Care Inventory" provide ways to track physical or mental health problems and organize important medical information.

Taking responsibility for good self-care is an important component to ensuring future success.

Holidays, in particular, often bring associations with addictive and unhealthy behaviors inconsistent with recovery. Engaging in appropriate, relaxing activities offers participants opportunities to begin to develop their own reservoir of happy memories associated with dates and seasons that previously created additional burdens.

We find that each holiday provides opportunities to develop new associations that are pleasurable, enjoyable and congruent with recovery. One example of that is St. Patrick's Day. Our activity of having each participant identify a "Hope or Dream" to display on a four-leaf clover provides a visual and emotional shift away from the common theme of drinking alcohol. This redirection of expectations was accepted without question. Some participants were not aware of the tradition of expressing wishes and dreams on St. Patrick's Day. Our hope is that a new association will come to participants later, emerging at a time that will help them or someone else lead a happier and more fulfilled life.

Kay: It is an adage in addiction work that holidays can be triggers. Anniversaries or special celebration days can make people in the early stages of recovery restless, irritable, and discontent. Roxanna and I enjoyed the challenge of finding activities that would not only take people's minds off being in rehab on a holiday but also provide lessons in managing the stressors. Verbalizing sad thoughts or uncomfortable emotions on Christmas Eve, Mother's Day, or Valentine's Day help individuals realize they are not alone in their feelings. And working on positive adaptations and alternative activities give clients a sense of mastery.

Roxanna: A poignant case was one of very low functioning woman who had spent much of her life, both as a child and as an adult, as homeless. At various times, social service workers had facilitated her securing a birth certificate, social security card, and other documents that would allow her to receive needed benefits. When she was admitted to the substance abuse program, she had lost track of these documents, thus significantly limiting her access to services.

It was with her in mind that I developed "Personal Portfolio," which teaches participants how to construct a secure folder out of a plain, donated grocery bag. The group embraced the activity as many had strong feelings about their own needs for a way to hold onto documents.

I do not know what became of the woman who inspired this activity. Others have given me feedback about how this simple technique made a profound difference and changed their perspective on their ability to manage their paperwork. Several participants, after a two-year follow up, indicated they were still using the folder they had created.

"Don't let shortsightedness interfere with your best vision of your future."

R oxanna E rickson-K lein

Calendar for the New Year

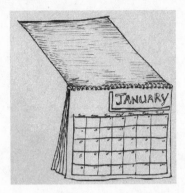

Location: Indoors

Time: 60 minutes

Materials: Copies of calendar pages for every month

Two pieces of stiff cardboard (two per person)

Ribbon or string

Markers or pens

Scissors

Hole punch

Glue or glue sticks

Variety of stickers or blank labels

Optional: fabric, craft paper, or other art supplies

Objectives

- To encourage the idea of self-responsibility for appointments, goal-setting, and planning ahead.

- To construct a tool that can support recovery by documenting important events in life and what has been accomplished.

Directions

1. Prepare the following before the session begins:

   A. Collect enough materials for every person in the group to make a calendar.

   B. Print or copy calendar pages for each participant. There are many websites that have a variety of free calendar formats. You might decide to have different pages to choose; to include some blank copies of "To Do" lists or "Goals for This Month"; or to make copies of some positive affirmations or recovery slogans for people to incorporate.

3. Instruct participants to choose 12 calendar pages and 2 pieces of cardboard for the cover.

4. Have them cut ribbon or string that will be used to tie the calendar together.

5. Direct participants to trim the calendar pages and the cover. They should leave an edge of about three-quarters of an inch, so they can place holes for the ribbon or string. All the calendar pages should be the same size, but the covers should be slightly bigger than the pages.

6. Punch holes in every page.

7. Tell participants to line up the holes and thread ribbon or string through the entire stack. After threading, have them tie a knot on each end.

8. Remind them to decorate the covers and the individual pages as desired.

9. Instruct them to add any important appointments or dates that they have coming up. Add reminders for each month, such as going to meetings, calling sponsor, seeing a doctor, or going to aftercare meetings.

Observations

This activity can be done at any time but makes a good start to organizing a new year. Early recovery can be a confusing time for people, and often executive function skills are poor. This activity encourages discussion about effective time management and follow-through. Successful people plan ahead. The groups appreciated the calendars and saw this as a small step in taking charge of one's life by writing down commitments.

Inspired by: Requests from clients for blank calendars on which to record their appointments.

January 2012

Sunday	Monday	Tuesday	Wednesday	Thursday	Friday	Saturday
1 New Year's Day *Always do your BEST*	2 *Be Cheerful*	3 *Use a Todo list*	4 *Don't worry*	5 *Pick up Trash*	6 *Be Kind*	7 *Help Others*
8 *Be honest*	9 *Remember your Beautiful*	10 *Expect a Miracle*	11 *Don't assume Anything*	12 *Believe in yourself*	13 *Enjoy New Things*	14 *Rest & Relax*
15 *Remember your victories*	16 ML King Jr. Day *Have accomplishments*	17 *Motivate yourself*	18 *Use your talents*	19 *Become a Champion*	20 *Have Fun*	21 *Finish Strong*
22 *Enjoy Church*	23 *Share good news*	24 *Always take action*	25 *Call a friend*	26 *My friend Terri's B-day*	27 *Creation not competition*	28 *Read*
29 *Ask Questions*	30 *Planners Win*	31 *Dream Big!*				

One participant gave herself positive affirmations and suggestions to maintian recovery on a daily basis, such as "Help Others, Expect a Miracle, Be Honest and Remember You're Beautiful."

Celebration for Recovery

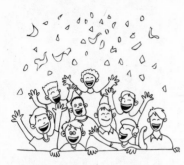

Location: Indoors

Time: 90 minutes

Materials: Writing paper

Poster paper

Colored construction paper

Pens, markers, or crayons

Collage materials

Celebration for Recovery Handout (one per person)

Optional: decorative art supplies

Objectives

- To have individuals in early recovery visualize having a sober party or other get-together at a future date.

- To consider the specific details of actually having sober fun and to anticipate future success on anniversary dates.

Directions

1. Divide participants into four groups. Each group will choose one time frame:

   - 1 week in recovery

   - 1 month in recovery

   - 1 year in recovery

   - 25 years in recovery

2. Tell groups to imagine they are planning a celebration for their assigned time frame.

3. Have each group discuss the questions on the Celebration for Recovery Handout and come up with creative ideas for the celebration. One person from each group should take notes.

4. Have each group create an invitation for the planned celebration. This can be a poster, a flyer, a card, a party invitation, or an advertisement. It should include as many imaginary details as possible, such as date, time, theme, menu, dress, rules, entertainment, or planned activities.

5. Allow about 30–40 minutes for the discussion and creation of the invitation.

6. Meet again as one group and have each small group present their ideas and invitations.

Observations

This activity was completed with enthusiasm, and posters and flyers were very creative. Having the clients actually think through concrete details of planning a sober get-together was helpful for them and made the concept workable. The only problem we found was that once the invitations were put up for others to see, people actually thought the events were real and wanted to go!

Inspired by: Clients' difficulties and limitations associated with envisioning a long-term, healthy future.

Celebration for Recovery HANDOUT

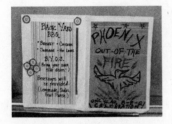

An invitation to a Back Yard BBQ celebrating one year of sobriety. The theme is "Phoenix Out of the Fire."

As a group, discuss the questions below and come up with ideas. Have one person take notes. Once you have answered all these questions, start to make an actual invitation to invite others to your celebration. It can be in the form of a poster, flyer, card, party invitation, or advertisement. It should include as many details as possible, such as date, time, theme, menu, dress, rules, cost, entertainment, or activities planned.

Plan Your Celebration

What would the celebration look like?

Who would be at the celebration (friends, relatives, adults, other people in recovery, children, dates, or families)?

What kind of clothes would you wear (dressy, formal, casual, costume party, or pajamas)?

What would be the theme (surprise, birthdays, private, big bash, supporting the homeless, costume party, or pajama party)?

What would you eat? Plan out the full menu.

What kind of beverages would be served? Plan for all participants.

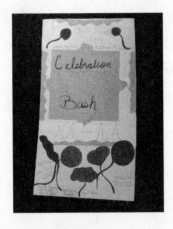

A one-month clean "Celebration Bash" for NA and AA attendees.

What would you do for entertainment? What if money is no object? What if you're on a budget?

Would this be free or would some or all people donate?

How much fun would this be for you? For others?

What gives this activity value?

Now you're ready to make your invitation!

"To become whole, to be in harmony, to be centered, to find one's true self, to be at peace with yourself, and the world—all of these are manifestations of healing."

RUBIN BATTINO

Easter Egg Affirmations

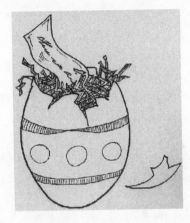

Location: Indoors or Outdoors

Time: 90 minutes

Materials: Plastic Easter eggs

Markers or pens

Small, wrapped candies (mints, chocolate eggs)

Paper

Copies of Affirmations

Scissors

Objectives

- To provide a positive and reinforcing activity for clients who are in residential treatment over a holiday.

- To show the utility of positive affirmations.

- To engage in planning and preparing for an activity that benefits others.

Directions

1. Discuss the Easter holiday in general terms. Some clients may miss children, some may miss family, or some may grieve losses from their childhood.

2. Continue with a short discussion about affirmations and the benefits of keeping a positive frame of mind. Give examples.

3. Explain that later in the day there will be an Easter egg hunt.

4. Fill each plastic egg with small pieces of candy and an affirmation. Encourage original and handwritten affirmations. For those who find this too difficult, provide them with affirmations that can be copied and cut in small strips.

Observations

Holidays are often a time of self-reflection or sadness, and sometimes a relapse trigger for inpatient clients. This activity was enjoyed by all participants, and they liked creating something for others. On one occasion, children at the treatment facility unexpectedly collected the eggs, and the clients delighted in this surprise turn of events.

Inspired by: Traditional Easter egg hunts.

"Being in recovery demands
change within our self. With
every change, something better
always comes along."

Pennie Johnson Carnes

Future You

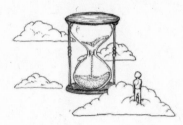

Location: Indoors

Time: 60–90 minutes

Materials: Writing paper

Pens, pencils, or markers

Cardstock or poster board

Future You Handout (one per person)

Optional: Decorative materials

Objectives

- To envision a positive future.

- To demonstrate how to set goals for the future and to think beyond current problems.

- To use Motivational Interviewing (MI) and Solution-Focused techniques to help clients articulate their personal values and goals.

Directions

1. Copy the Future You Handouts, putting a date two years from the date of the activity.

2. Promote a discussion about how and why we might want to set goals for the future. We know that people who write about their personal goals are more likely to achieve them. Those who can imagine a positive future for themselves tend to be happier and have less stress.

3. Ask participants to think about personal values and goals, using questions such as, *What is important? How will you know when your problems are no longer present? What will life look like?*

4. Have participants imagine life two years from the present time.

5. Using the Future You Handout, have each person jot down some ideas and answers to the questions. Encourage them to be as specific as possible.

6. After everyone has made some notes, have them transfer these ideas to writing paper or poster board. Words or drawings may be used.

Observations

It was difficult for many individuals to come up with concrete ideas for what their life would look like. It is important to encourage participants to be as specific as possible, for example, if having a job is part of the plan, what kind of job? Full-time or part-time? Where will it be located? Making some notes *before* they start the project works much better. Motivational Interviewing and Solution-Focused techniques can be effectively adapted to this activity, for example, what will your future look like? Are your future goals consistent with current behaviors? Teaching participants to refocus their time perspective from negative thoughts about the past into more productive, positive pathways for the future will produce better outcomes and will lessen stress and PTSD symptoms.

Inspired by: The book, *Time Cure: Overcoming PTSD with the New Psychology of Time Perspective Therapy,* by Philip Zimbardo, PhD, Richard Sword, PhD, and Rosemary Sword (Jossey-Bass, 2012).

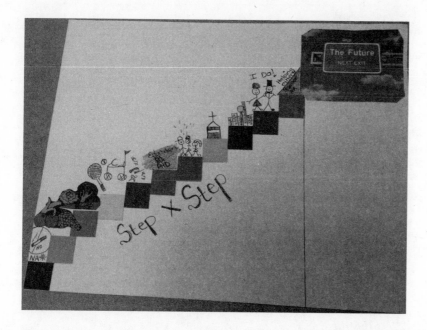

This person envisioned the following steps of her recovery into the future: stopping smoking, eating healthy, exercising regularly, getting a job, getting her education, having a family, going to church, belonging to the community, getting married, and helping others as a NA sponsor.

Future You HANDOUT

What will my life look like on _____ (fill in a future date two years from now).

Where will I be and what will I be doing?

Setting positive goals for yourself for the future is important. People who write about their personal goals are more likely to achieve them. Also, people who can imagine a positive future for themselves tend to be happier and have less stress. Research has shown that when people refocus their time perspective from negative thoughts about the past into more productive, positive pathways for the future, their quality of life and mental functioning improves.

DIRECTIONS

Write in detail what your life will look like two years from today. You can use words or pictures.

What will you being doing two years from now? Try to envision an ideal future. What are your personal dreams today? Imagine who you want to be.

Where are you living?   Who are you living with?
What do you look like?   How busy is your day?
How do you behave with others?   What are your relationships like?

What are you passionate about?
How do you make time or money for the things you love to do?

All the areas of your life should be included within your plan:

Career, Job   Hobbies
Friends   Recreation
Family   Exercise
Physical Environment   Recovery
Health   Goals
Education   Money
Personal Growth   Fun

"The success of any method derives from its capacity to join and empower the client's reality."

Stephen Gilligan

Give Yourself a Checkup

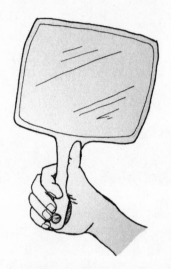

Location: Indoors

Time: 45 minutes

Materials: Give Yourself a Checkup Handout, (4 per person)

Current Medicine Log (4 per person)

Objectives

- To teach participants to self-assess their own health status and provide a measure that can be looked at periodically.

- To encourage self-advocacy of healthcare needs.

Directions

1. Distribute Give Yourself a Checkup Handouts and encourage participants to reflect upon their current health as they answer each of the questions.

2. Give participants several extra blank forms to complete in thirty days, and periodically thereafter, to provide an objective tool by which they can assess their own well-being.

3. Stress that while some conditions need immediate attention, often it is helpful to chart trends in one's health and share them with physicians and other healthcare providers.

4. If anyone has questions about a medical condition or wants additional information, remind them to talk with medical personnel on campus or with his or her doctor.

5. Pass out the Current Medicine Log and give participants time to fill it out completely. Stress the importance of keeping a current medication list in their purse or wallet.

6. Instruct participants to keep all forms for their own self-evaluation.

Observations

These forms were used in several groups ranging in size from eight to fifteen. The forms were effective in calling attention to participants' centrally important indicators of health. Participants were not encouraged to share their findings but rather to take the information seriously and to follow-up as they saw fit. Several participants remarked that they always had a new doctor each time they went in for medications, but few had considered monitoring their own health to be important. Overall, this is an important step in accepting responsibility for one's healthcare.

Inspired by: Roxanna's years of work in healthcare and observations on how ill-equipped many people are in monitoring their own health needs.

Give Yourself a Checkup HANDOUT

Name _____ Date _____

Circle your answers. Answer as best you can.

Do you have any special health needs right now?   YES   NO

If YES, what are they: _____

_____

1. How healthy do you feel RIGHT NOW?

   1   2   3   4   5   6   7   8   9   10
   Sick   Average health   Completely well

2. How healthy have you been feeling THIS WEEK?

   1   2   3   4   5   6   7   8   9   10
   Sick   Average health   Completely well

3. How is your feeling of well-being as compared to LAST WEEK?

   1   2   3   4   5   6   7   8   9   10
   Sick   Average health   Completely well

4. How is your feeling of well-being as compared to LAST MONTH?

   1   2   3   4   5   6   7   8   9   10
   Much worse   The same   Much better

5. If you take medication, do you take it regularly?

                   Yes   No   Sometimes

6. Do you know the names and doses of your medications?

        I know them all.   I know some of them.   I have no idea.

7. What is your technique for remembering to take medications (example: med box)?

   _____

8. Do you take your medications when you are supposed to?

   I always remember to take my meds.   I often don't take my meds on time.

9. Are you able to stay on track about time, place, schedule, or responsibilities?

                   Yes   No   Sometimes

10. Are you able to read a short article that is interesting?

                              Yes   No   Sometimes

11. Can you follow a conversation?

                                Yes   No   Sometimes

12. Do you have unusual ideas, including intrusive thoughts, hallucinations, voices, shadows, feelings, or get stuck with repetition of ideas?

                                Yes   No   Sometimes

13. Have you noticed changes in your judgment lately?

I always do what's right.   I sometimes make big mistakes.   I often make big mistakes.

14. How is your impulse control?

I have no patience.   I sometimes have patience.   I'm willing to work hard for rewards later.

15. How are you emotionally?

        Mostly sad   Sometimes sad, sometimes happy   Mostly happy

16. How is your activity level?

                    Low energy   Average energy   Lots of energy

17. How is your appetite?

      Never hungry   Normal hunger at meal times   Really hungry most of the time

18. About how many hours of sleep are you getting at night? _____

Here is an example of how to fill out the Current Medicine Log.

NAME OF MEDICATION & STRENGTH
Lisinopril HCTZ
10 mg tablets

WHAT'S IT FOR
blood pressure

DOSE, HOW OFTEN
2 tablets (20 mg) two times a day (but I ran out last week)

PRESCRIBING DR.
Smith at Metrocare

REFILL DATE
October 25, 2013

WHEN STARTED / LAST TIME DOSE CHANGED
started about 5 years ago and increased to 2 times a day last month

REASON FOR CHANGE
increased because my blood pressure was high

CURRENT MEDICINE LOG

(Keep all old sheets in your medical records.)

TODAY'S DATE _____

NAME OF MEDICATION & STRENGTH	WHAT'S IT FOR	DOSE, HOW OFTEN	PRESCRIBING DR.	REFILL DATE	WHEN STARTED / LAST TIME THE DOSE CHANGED	REASON FOR CHANGE

ALLERGIES TO MEDICINES:

"Healthy growth requires a
balance of successful learning,
nourishment, rest, and self-care."

Roxanna Erickson-Klein

Goal Boards

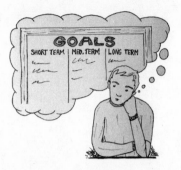

Location: Indoors

Time: 90 minutes

Materials: Pieces of cardboard or foam board (about 24" long and 10" high)

Colored marker

Rulers

Goal Boards Handout (one per person)

Objectives

- To imagine in concrete terms what positive change in life can look like.

- To teach the benefits of planning and prioritizing and breaking larger tasks into small steps that can be accomplished.

Directions

1. Prepare a sample goal board in advance. Goals provide direction and purpose to life and help us make good decisions. This activity will help participants think about priorities and how to achieve them successfully. It will increase participants' chances of meeting basic needs as well as envisioning dreams for the future. Writing down goals and looking at them frequently will make someone more likely to achieve them.

2. Begin a discussion about goals. Read aloud the following:

   There are different kinds of goals in life: short-term (immediate), medium-term (in the next few months), and long-term (in several years). There are areas in life in which it might be helpful to set goals, such as employment, education, housing, financial independence, child custody, or fitness. Be specific and look at all the small steps that may be required. For example, "getting a job" might entail writing a resume (short-term), attending job training, applying for employment (medium-term), and then finding your dream job (long-term). Goals should be realistic, positive, and focus on performance instead of outcome. Creating a goal board can help you achieve clarity and can also be used for personal accountability.

3. Ask each participant to take a long sheet of card stock or foam board.

4. Pass out the Goal Boards Handout. Direct participants to draw three columns with the headings: Short-Term Goals, Medium-Term Goals, Long-Term Goals

5. Have participants choose three or four areas in their life where they would like to have positive change.

6. Tell participants that each column should be filled in with the steps that would realistically be taken to achieve the goal.

7. Invite participants to share their goal boards with the group.

Observations

This activity works best with a smaller group of approximately six to ten people so that the facilitator can provide guidance and encouragement. When done with a group of thirty, meaningful planning could not be attained. Many participants needed assistance coming up with concrete steps to reach future goals, but they were enthusiastic about the finished boards.

Inspired by: A doctoral intern at Nexus, Kari L.

Goal Boards HANDOUT

What areas in your life would you like to have positive change?

employment

career

education

housing

financial independence

family

child custody

physical fitness

physical health

mental health

spiritual or ethical

other area

Make three columns on your paper. Label the first Short-Term Goals, the second Medium-Term Goals, and the last Long-Term Goals. Now choose three or four areas where you would like to make a positive change (see list above for suggestions).

You may want to start with Long-Term Goals (several years from now) and work backward. Or, you may start with your immediate Short-Term Goals, such as "get housing." Be as specific as possible.

Under each goal, write any practical steps you will need to take to achieve it. What is the first thing you will have to do? The next thing?

"Everyone has the capacity for positive change. And people are their own agents of change. Envision your change now."

KAY COLBERT

Holiday Hands

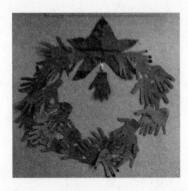

Location: Indoors

Time: 60 minutes

Materials: Construction paper (colors symbolic of the holiday)

Markers

Large surface for display, such as windows, sliding glass doors, or a wall

Tape or glue dots

Optional: Other decorative supplies

Objectives

- To recognize the holidays in a participatory manner.
- To create an engaging activity that can be done with any number of people.

Directions

1. Make the following preparations before the session begins:

    A. Select a design that is representative of the upcoming holiday.

    B. If any additional pieces are needed to complete the display, prepare them from poster board. For example, a star would accent a Christmas tree, a red bow for a wreath, or green stem to add to a pumpkin.

    C. Identify a display area, and if possible, choose an area where participants can post their own contributions as they complete them.

    D. Trace and cut sample hands on colored paper.

5. Explain the process and show the sample hands.

6. Pass out colored construction paper that matches the theme. Provide two pages per participant.

7. Invite participants to trace one hand on one piece of paper. Then have them ask another group member to trace his or her other hand on the second piece of construction paper.

8. Instruct participants to cut, decorate, and sign or date their hand tracings, as desired.

9. Post the hands, once finished, to form the holiday shape. Have one person oversee the process of forming the hands into the shape.

Observations

This activity works very well in large groups. On each of the occasions it was tried, two participants volunteered to oversee the artistic posting of the hands. The activity was done twice for Christmas, once on the Fourth of July, and twice for Halloween. On each occasion, the activity was followed with extensive processing of feelings of gratitude for acknowledgment of the holiday and the sense of inclusion in a celebration. For Christmas, green was used; both a wreath and a tree were formed on windows in a group room. For the Fourth of July, participants chose red, white, or blue, and hands were arranged on a bulletin board to construct a flag. The orange hands on Halloween formed a happy jack-o'-lantern.

Inspired by: This is a long-standing family tradition for Roxanna in which hands are traced yearly, autographed, dated, and then arranged for holiday decorations that also illustrate the growth and development of children in the family.

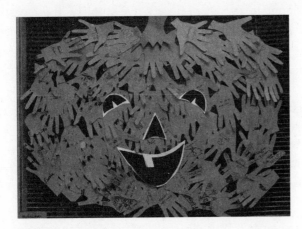

A completed jack-o'-lantern.

July Fourth Freedom Poems

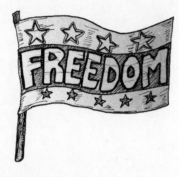

Location: Indoors or Outdoors

Time: 60 minutes

Materials: July Fourth Freedom Poems Handout (one per person)

Objectives

- To compare the freedom often talked about on the Fourth of July with personal freedom from alcohol and other drugs or other addictive behaviors.

Directions

1. Hold a brief discussion about the history of Independence Day in the United States.

2. Ask about different meanings for the words "freedom" or "independence."

3. Have participants discuss how these ideas can apply to their own personal experiences.

4. Pass out the July Fourth Freedom Poems Handout to each participant.

5. Ask volunteers to read their poems aloud.

Observations

This was done in a group of twenty-five to thirty. Those participants with fewer literacy skills needed some assistance with writing, but everyone participated actively. The sharing of the finished poems was heartfelt.

Inspired by: Materials for classroom teachers that encourage creating poems from templates.

July Fourth Freedom Poems HANDOUT

Fill in the blanks to create your independence story.

FREEDOM FOR ME IS _____ AND _____

I DREAM OF _____

NOW I NOTICE _____

NOW I HEAR _____

NOW I SEE _____

NOW I SAY _____

NOW I AM _____

I AM FEELING _____

I AM GOOD AT _____

I AM WORKING TO _____

NOW I HOPE _____

I AM CHANGING _____

I AM BECOMING _____

I WILL LEAVE BEHIND _____

I AM GETTING BETTER AT _____

I HAVE ALREADY LEARNED HOW TO _____

A CHANGE IN ME IS _____

I WILL BE _____

I WILL REMIND MYSELF _____

YOU WILL SEE CHANGE IN MY _____

I WILL WALK WITH _____

I WILL TALK WITH _____

I WILL SING WITH _____

INDEPENDENCE FOR ME TODAY IS _____

Mother's Day Flower Garden

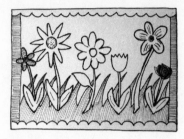

Location: Indoors

Time: 60 minutes

Materials: Sample cutouts or illustrations of flowers

Scissors

Glue

Colored Paper

Markers

Bulletin board

Tacks

Objectives

- To work together to construct a feeling of appreciation and beauty for a holiday that can be particularly difficult for many in recovery.

Directions

1. Discuss the meaning of Mother's Day and encourage participants to express true feelings of loss and frustration or of appreciation and love.

2. Encourage collaboration on a public bulletin board as one means of showing how working together can sometimes soothe painful feelings, as well as providing relaxation.

3. Identify a theme for the bulletin board, such as a "Garden of Love and Appreciation," and encourage participants to use their imagination to generate floral images.

4. Invite participants to show their work and express the meaning behind it to the larger group.

Observations

This bulletin board project was one of a series of seasonal and open group activities that decorated a large space in a public area. In this activity, the discussion revealed considerable shame and guilt from many participants that was associated with not having a mother who cared for them. For women who were mothers themselves, there was the additional thought that they had not been the type of mother they wanted to be for their children. Some mothers were separated from their children permanently, and this created regret and painful feelings. The discussion seemed to be quite useful as it addressed common themes associated with substance abuse. The participants had little difficulty in providing support and empathy for one another and were encouraging about expressing those feelings in a beautiful way. A few chose to use their materials to construct cards, some to themselves.

It was helpful to have the bulletin board close at hand where the participants could add to the blossoming garden after their work was completed. The sample was a size and shape that worked well within the space available, though there were no limits placed on the construction.

This activity can be adapted for Father's Day. Instead of floral images, participants can make examples of times or activities spent with a dad or being a dad themselves. The garden background can be used, or an alternative idea is a road map and images can be signposts along the way.

Inspired by: Awareness that holidays, and Mother's Day in a very intimate way, are particularly challenging for people in institutional settings.

Personal Portfolios

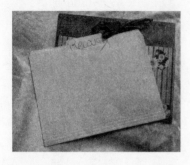

Location: Indoors

Time: 90 minutes

Materials: Personal Portfolio Handouts (one per person)

Clock with secondhand

Paper grocery bags (one per person, preferably with handles)

Manila folders (one or more per person)

Large construction paper

Notebook paper (about five sheets per person)

Markers

Ribbons

Optional: Decorating supplies

Objectives

- To illustrate the value of a systematic approach to managing responsibilities.

- To give the opportunity to construct a personal portfolio.

Directions

1. Prepare the following before the session:

   A. Make a sample portfolio for viewing.

   B. Copy instruction sheets for each participant.

   C. Prepare warm-up activity materials.

4. Have participants complete the warm-up activity before portfolios are started, using the Personal Portfolio Handouts.

   A. Pass out the first handout page with scattered numbers—FACE DOWN.

   B. Instruct the group to circle the numbers in sequential order: 1, 2 . . .

   C. Have the participants turn over the page and begin circling.

   D. Time the participants for one minute. At the end of one minute, ask them to stop.

   E. Pass out the second handout page with numbers in quadrants—FACE DOWN.

   F. Instruct the group to look in quadrants A, B, C, D, then A . . .

   G. Have the participants turn over the page and begin circling.

   H. Time the participants for one minute. At the end of one minute, ask them to stop.

   I. Facilitate group discussion on the differences in finding the numbers that were organized in a systematic way versus a random way.

10. Pass out materials, including notebook paper and single manila folders.

11. Encourage each participant to envision his or her own list of needed files. Allow 5 to 10 minutes to write the list.

12. Ask volunteers to share their list of planned files with group.

13. Distribute instructions and materials to compile own portfolio. Allow 40 minutes for work time.

14. Elicit group feedback regarding choices made and perceived utility of the activity.

Observations

The warm-up activity vividly illustrated the efficiency of having a systematic method of attending to matters. By participating in the choice of how to label the internal folders, individuals have already begun the process of applying the principles to personal life situations. The first time this activity was done in a group of thirty-five with two facilitators. Pre-made folio covers were used, standard manila file folders were provided, and the activity was done in one hour. The participants found the activity so helpful that a second run was done using grocery sacks that the women were encouraged to cut into appropriate shapes and decorate.

Feedback was positive and enthusiastic regarding the practical approach to managing legal papers, housing information, twelve-step exercises, and other materials with which numerous participants had struggled. Individual decision-making regarding file folder contents facilitates personal investment and tailoring to personal needs.

Several clients later told us that this activity was an important and memorable step in their recovery.

Inspired by: The warm-up activity was done in a college course. Many other resources and personal experiences promote file folder systems of organizing and prioritizing. This activity was conceptualized after noting the difficulties of individual clients in holding onto personal valuables, including such essentials as birth certificates.

Personal Portfolios HANDOUT

Circle the Numbers

This is a timed activity. You will be timed for one minute.

Counting in order, circle as many numbers as you can.

1   13   26   2
    41   18
        5   14   30
37   33
    21   42   46
9   25   6   38   22
    49   45
29   50
        17   34   10

40   31
    8   12   47   27

16   32   7   15
    48   23

        28   35   39
44   43
    20

4   24   36   11   19   3

Personal Portfolios HANDOUT

Circle the Numbers

This is a timed activity. You will be timed for one minute.

Counting in order, circle as many numbers as you can.

1   13   26   2
41   18
5   14   30
37   33
21   42   46
9   25   6   38   22
49   45
29   17   34   10   50

40   31
8   12   47   27
16   48   32   7   15
23
28   35   39
44   43
20
4   24   36   11   19   3

Personal Portfolios HANDOUT

Turn a Grocery Bag into a Portfolio

1. Locate a full-size standard grocery bag from a store; handles add a nice feature.

2. Open the bag and stand it on the table in front of you.

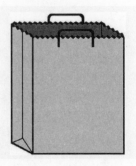

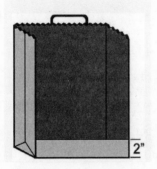

3. Cut the corner seams on each side of the front, starting at the top corner and ending about two inches from the bottom.

4. Fold the front flap forward, cut the bottom edge off, and throw it away. This will leave a bag that has three tall sides and one short side.

5. Fold up the bottom and flatten it. This creates a flat bag with a pocket at the bottom.

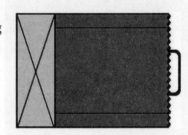

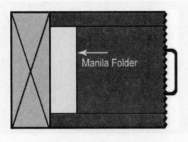

6. Insert a standard manila folder into the pocket.

7. Fold the top of the bag over the manila folder to form a closed wallet.

8. Secure with ribbon or string.

9. Decorate as desired.

10. Construct additional interior folders with colored manila paper.

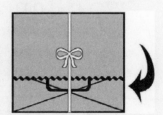

"Be kind to yourself. Allow others to help you. Expect the miracles of change."

PENNIE JOHNSON CARNES

Pick a Holiday

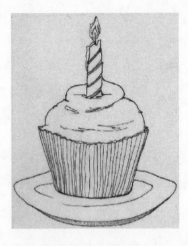

Location: Indoors

Time: 60–90 minutes

Materials: Pick a Holiday Handout (one per person)

Colored paper

Markers or crayons

Glue

Scissors

Optional: Magazines

Objectives

- To raise awareness of individual vulnerability to relapse around holidays.

- To imagine oneself successfully participating in recovery during a time that has been problematic.

- To develop strategies and ideas that will allow for self-instruction during vulnerable times.

Directions

1. Discuss the vulnerability that some people have in relapsing around a holiday.

2. Invite participants to identify one or more holidays that are difficult for them.

3. Provide Pick a Holiday Handouts and art supplies so that individuals can write about and illustrate their own image of safely making it through a potentially difficult interval of time.

4. Allow about 40 minutes for individual decision making and art compositions.

5. Convene in a setting where the participants can show their creation to the group.

6. Invite participants to stand before the group and talk about their experience with this activity.

Observations

The vast majority of the participants wanted to discuss their creation. The holidays ranged from Mother's and Father's Day, Thanksgiving, St. Patrick's Day, Mardi Gras—even President's Day and the Super Bowl were represented. The most commonly represented holidays were Valentine's Day, Christmas, Mother's Day, and birthdays (of their own or their children). The creative directions to approach this task were varied and unique. This activity proved to be one of the most powerful of any included in this collection with participants telling about painful associations and relapse triggers that have been problematic in the past. Many were openly emotional and tearful and expressed hope that this activity will help them maintain recovery.

Inspired by: Recognition of how challenging holidays and celebrations can be for people in early recovery.

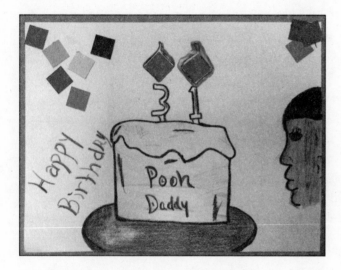

A client's self-portrait of her next birthday.

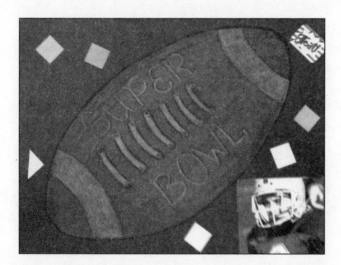

Super Bowl celebrations are challenging for one person.

Pick a Holiday HANDOUT

Holidays are often associated with relapse. Reasons for this are many:

- Sometimes it is the way that people are used to celebrating with their friends or family.

- Sometimes people want to forget about things.

- Sometimes people don't know what to do with the extra, flexible time.

- Sometimes people feel depressed or lonely and want to numb that feeling.

- Sometimes there are painful memories of when you missed a holiday or event because of your drinking or using.

- And sometimes people get caught up in plans that someone else has made.

The purpose of this activity is to raise awareness that holidays are high-risk times for relapse. By thinking about risks in advance, you can better prepare and protect yourself from relapse.

Think about a holiday at any time of the year that presents the greatest risk to you. Use the art materials to create an image of a holiday. Envision a strong, healthy time in which you are not vulnerable to using substances. EVEN if the holiday is traditionally associated with substance use, such as St. Patrick's Day or Mardi Gras, think about celebrating in a safe, responsible way that supports recovery. Do not limit yourself to national holidays; think about your own family and cultural traditions.

It can be a time that is traditionally happy.

Birthdays	Graduations	Super Bowl

Or events that are sad.

Funerals	Anniversary of a death, departure, or loss

Or it can be a regularly observed holiday.

New Year's Eve	Independence Day	Chanukah
Valentine's Day	Easter	Halloween
Mardi Gras	Passover	Thanksgiving
St. Patrick's Day	Christmas	Groundhog Day
April Fool's Day	Veterans Day	Labor Day
Earth Day	Mother's Day	Father's Day
Cinco de Mayo	Diwali	Ramadan

"The inner child within us has the answers you are seeking. Allow him or her to play with these exercises and speak to your heart and mind."

PENNIE JOHNSON CARNES

Recovery Pumpkins

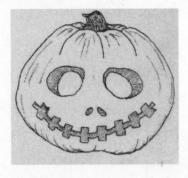

Objectives

- To provide a fall celebration that is focused on recovery-related issues.
- To turn to expressive art during a holiday that otherwise may be particularly difficult.

Directions

1. Distribute a pumpkin to each participant.

2. Inform participants that the pumpkins will be decorated, not carved.

3. Have participants select one the following categories for their pumpkin (judging or competition can be optional):

   A. Recovery Pumpkin—How can you decorate to illustrate being in recovery?

   B. Family Pumpkin—It may be silly or scary, but what will your family pumpkin look like?

   C. Pumpkin of the Future—What does the future hold, even for a jack-o'-lantern?

   D. Most Creative—Let your creativity shine here, anything goes.

5. Have participants display their pumpkin and award a small prize to the top three winners in each category. Peers can vote for the winners, or staff can choose.

Location: Indoors or Outdoors

Time: 90 minutes

Materials: Small pumpkins (one per person)

Colored markers, paint pens, or fabric paint

Craft supplies (glitter, sequins, yarn, or collage materials)

Small blank note cards

Small prizes for each winner

Optional: Miniature pumpkins or gourds

Observations

The group atmosphere was congenial as participants worked on the pumpkins. The treatment center had an organic garden where the clients grew pumpkins, so it was especially satisfying for them to pick, decorate, and display them. Bags of miniature pumpkins were also purchased and decorated with paint and yarn. It made the holiday positive, especially for clients who missed their children and the opportunity to take them trick-or-treating. Some clients made extra pumpkins to give to their children or a relative. Many said they were inspired to do this activity with their children next year.

Inspired by: Adapted from a suggestion by a fellow staff member.

Self-Care Inventory

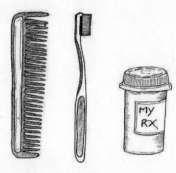

Location: Indoors or Outdoors

Time: 60 minutes

Materials: Pens or pencils

Self-Care Inventory Handout (one per person)

Objectives

- To nurture a growing awareness of the elements of responsible self-care.

Directions

1. Divide group into four smaller groups.

2. Assign each of the four groups one of the following topics to present: Spiritual Centering, Body Health, Social Connections and Family Life, and Mental Health.

3. Ask each group to discuss the ways in which each question under its topic is related to recovery. Groups come up with key points, tips, suggestions, or advice. Give groups 20 minutes to discuss and prepare for the next step.

4. Have each group present its topic to the larger audience. Each group needs to decide if there will be a spokesperson or the whole group will take turns presenting. The presentation should last about 5 minutes.

5. At the end of each presentation, encourage the whole group to ask questions or add to the points made by the presenters.

Observations

This activity was done twice, each time with a large group of forty. Most, though not all, of the presentations were done with all group members having a role in the presentation. The style ranged from didactic to a series of skits in which various elements of the topic were addressed in a humorous way. Perhaps the most important aspect of this activity is to call attention to what is not being addressed in various participants' lives. Most participants appreciated the opportunity to offer information to the larger group. Presentations were consistently well thought out.

Inspired by: Work in healthcare settings.

Self-Care Inventory HANDOUT

Answer the questions below. Then discuss with your group members how each question in your topic is related to recovery.

Spiritual Centering

Do I have a sense of a larger purpose?

Do I have a fellowship of others with similar beliefs?

Do I set aside time for connecting with the beauty around me?

Am I at peace with my beliefs?

Body Health

Do I know how much sleep I need for good health?

Do I get the right number of hours of sleep if I average the week?

Am I able to fall asleep and stay asleep with reasonable ease?

Am I a healthy weight (body mass index)?

Do I eat fresh fruits or vegetables every day?

Do I eat for nutrition or for stress?

Does my body feel healthy?

Do I get a reasonable amount of exercise every week?

Do I see the dentist every year?

Do I go in for medical checkups?

Am I up-to-date with dental, medical, and other checkups?

Do I know the name of my doctor?

Do I schedule and keep track of my own appointments?

Do I know the names of my medicines?

Do I take my medicines as prescribed?

Do I know what the medicines are expected to do for me?

Social Connections and Family Life

Am I living rather independently given current circumstances?

Do I actively contribute to my household in tangible ways? (financial, work, social)

Do I give more than I take in?

Is my household or family life chaotic?

Do I bring beauty into my surroundings?

Do I have friends who I can trust?

Do I make time for my friends?

Do I know how to have fun with others in healthy ways?

Do I make an effort to make others happy?

Mental Health

Do I make time for myself?

Do I accept my limitations and also my strengths?

Is there beauty in my life?

Am I continuing to learn?

Do I forgive others and myself when a mistake is made?

Can I ask for help when I need it?

Do I express negative feelings in a healthy manner?

Is there music in my life?

Do I have healthy ways to relax?

Self-Watering Container Gardens

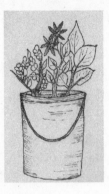

Location: Outdoors

Time: 25–30 minutes (depending on number of participants)

Materials: For each participant:

2 flexible clear plastic cups (when nested they need to have a gap of about 1 or 2 inches between the interior and exterior cup)

1 wide drinking straw

1 cup potting soil

1 or 2 seeds of sunflowers, black-eyed peas, or squash

Strip of cotton t-shirt or rag

Scissors

Water

Objectives

- To learn how to construct a simple, personal garden with a self-watering system.

Directions

1. Prepare a sample container with a sprouted seed. Most seeds will sprout within 3–7 days.

2. Assemble group outside, sitting at tables or in a circle on the ground. Explain that today's activity will involve construction of a small, individual container garden for each person. This method of gardening can be used to grow flowers or vegetables in a small space and is easy to maintain as it self-waters.

3. Using the inside cup, cut a section out of the bottom corner that is large enough to stick the straw through.

4. Cut the cotton cloth into a strip about 3 inches × 1 inch.

5. Stuff the cotton strip in the hole next to the straw, so that it holds the straw into place and reaches the bottom of the outside cup when the cups are nested.

6. Place the inside cup in the outside cup to see that the straw is positioned for refilling the water as needed. The cotton strip must be positioned so that it will wick water from the outside cup into the soil held in the inside cup.

7. Once the cutting is done, put some soil into the inside cup. Hold the cotton strip up so it reaches high near where the roots will be looking for water.

8. Put some water in the outside cup and nest the two cups.

9. Bury a seed a quarter of an inch into the soil.

10. Water lightly.

11. Place in the sun, and refill when the reservoir is low.

Observations

This activity was done in conjunction with a variety of outdoor activities and provided a "take home" reward as well as developing awareness of the simplicity of container gardening. The sunflower seeds sprouted well, and the participants cared for their plants until they left the facility. In hot weather, cups may need water every two to three days. Participants transplanted surviving seedlings into a larger garden area.

Inspired by: A Houston Food Bank project in which buckets and PVC pipes were used to construct container gardens. The food bank recipients successfully grow their own vegetables, including lettuce, carrots and tomatoes. The self-watering concept eliminates the need for daily watering, even in dry, hot weather.

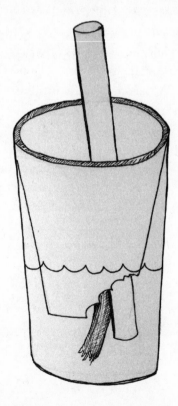

Cutaway diagram of a plastic cup used for a container.

St. Patrick's Day Hopes and Dreams

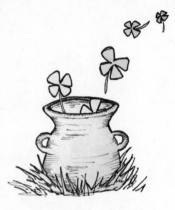

Objectives

- To redefine a holiday traditionally associated with alcohol consumption.

Directions

1. Prepare a public bulletin board with a rainbow and a black cauldron or pot of gold at the end of the rainbow.

2. Pass out clover templates or green paper to make clovers.

3. Encourage participants to identify their hopes and dreams and write their wishes on a clover.

4. Gather the clovers and arrange them as if they are coming out of the cauldron.

Observations

This activity was done with a large group concurrent with a free-art recreation time. A team of volunteers constructed the bulletin board using black paper plates to create the cauldron. We used die-cut clovers instead of cutting them by hand. The participants expressed much appreciation for the opportunity to adjust thinking about the holiday to a time to reflect on one's true values.

Inspired by: Watching the drinking at a St. Patrick's Day parade and recognizing the difficulties this holiday poses for those whom alcohol is problematic.

Location: Indoors

Time: 20–30 minutes

Materials: Public bulletin board

Black paper cauldron

Rainbow

Clover templates or green paper

Markers

Tacks

Optional: Scissors

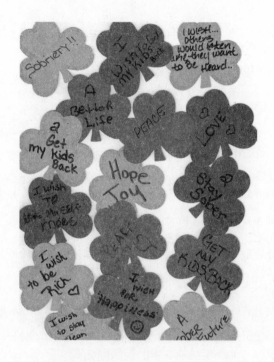

Examples of clover wishes.

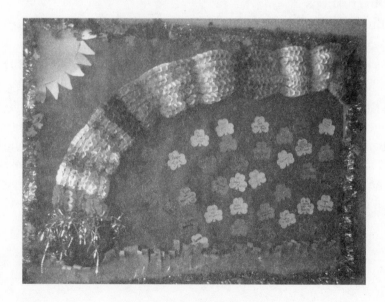

Completed bulletin board.

Thanksgiving Gratitude Turkey

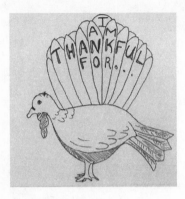

Location: Indoors

Time: 30 minutes

Materials: Public bulletin board

Tacks

Turkey image

Colored paper

Feather templates or feather shapes

Markers

Objectives

- To recognize the holiday in a traditional way while participating in healthy, positive self-reflection.

- To focus on moments of gratitude rather than resentments.

Directions

1. Find a bulletin board or other display area. Cover background of display area with plain colored paper. Place the body of the a turkey on the background.

2. Instruct participants to cut feathers from colored paper, by freehand, or by using templates.

3. Encourage participants to identify something they are grateful for this Thanksgiving.

4. Fan out the feathers to display the participants' messages.

5. Allow each participant to tell the group what his or her feather represents, or they can post it quietly without comment.

Observations

This activity was done with a large group concurrent with free recreation time. A team of volunteers constructed the bulletin board using a honeycomb pre-made turkey. It made a fun addition to the art as the participants were able to stick their feathers right on the turkey and remove them to read aloud. Every participant in this large group of forty wanted to tell the group what his or her feather represented. Several participants made more than one feather, and some of the feathers were very ornate. As participants stood before the group, ready to post their feathers, several became tearful, and all expressed gratitude for having the opportunity to come together in a safe place of recovery.

The second time this activity was done, a volunteer cut a turkey shape out of a brown grocery sack and put it on the bulletin board. Participants enjoyed the homemade turkey as much as the purchased one. In both cases, participants wrote simple personal messages of gratefulness on their feathers.

The Alcoholics Anonymous concept of gratitude in recovery may also be included as part of the discussion. Bill W. was a cofounder of Alcoholics Anonymous. In a piece titled, "What Is Acceptance?" from March 1962, he wrote about taking a full inventory of one's blessings, accepting the many gifts that are yours (both tangible and spiritual), and trying to achieve a state of joyful gratitude. The full text may be found online.

Inspired by: Elementary school projects with the positive focus on gratitude.

Valentine's Day Letter to Loved Ones

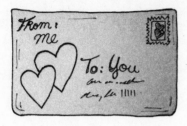

Location: Indoors

Time: 90 minutes

Materials: Colored paper

Glue or glue sticks

Scissors

Markers

Writing paper

Envelopes

Stamps

Objectives

- To acknowledge a holiday that is typically difficult for individuals in recovery and generate a proactive and positive response to the holiday.

- To support an ongoing sense of well-being by reciprocating positive deeds and positive feelings.

Directions

1. Discuss the upcoming Valentine's Day and invite participants to comment on their past experiences and how they might generate positive experiences for the holiday.

2. Suggest that this occasion presents the opportunity to recognize the loving influence of someone else.

3. Invite participants to use the supplies to construct a letter "to anyone you wish to brighten the day of," whether it be themselves, a friend, relative, past teacher, or anyone who has helped them feel special. The only restriction is that the letter needs to be positive.

4. On completion of the activity, invite participants to share their letters, including their experience of deciding whom to write.

5. Offer envelopes and stamps if participants wish to actually mail their letters.

Observations

It is a common experience for individuals to feel omitted or forgotten on Valentine's Day, even for those who are not in recovery. When encouraging participants to express emotions about the day, a common theme of feeling "left out" was dominant. Expression of this emotion brought about an awareness that others felt the same. Often individuals in recovery perceived that everyone else has a wonderful, intimate partner relationship to celebrate except them. They verbalized the fear they would never find love because of things done in the past. Or, they talked about remorse over past relationships damaged by addiction. To hear that others shared their feelings was very healing. The opportunity to reach out to someone else with a heartfelt letter was enthusiastically embraced. Almost 100 percent of the participants expressed an active desire to speak to the group and share the contents of their letters. The letters were written to a broad group of recipients including former teachers, neighbors, aunts, mothers, children, treatment center staff, individuals living or deceased, and to themselves.

Inspired by: Many tales of being lonely on Valentine's Day.

Appendix

A THE TWELVE STEPS OF ALCOHOLICS ANONYMOUS

1. We admitted we were powerless over alcohol—that our lives had become unmanageable.

2. Came to believe that a Power greater than ourselves could restore us to sanity.

3. Made a decision to turn our will and our lives over to the care of God *as we understood Him.*

4. Made a searching and fearless moral inventory of ourselves.

5. Admitted to God, to ourselves, and to another human being the exact nature of our wrongs.

6. Were entirely ready to have God remove all these defects of character.

7. Humbly asked Him to remove our shortcomings.

8. Made a list of all persons we had harmed, and became willing to make amends to them all.

9. Made direct amends to such people wherever possible, except when to do so would injure them or others.

10. Continued to take personal inventory and when we were wrong promptly admitted it.

11. Sought through prayer and meditation to improve our conscious contact with God, *as we understood Him*, praying only for knowledge of His will for us and the power to carry that out.

12. Having had a spiritual awakening as the result of these Steps, we tried to carry this message to alcoholics, and to practice these principles in all our affairs.

B   THE TWELVE STEPS OF NARCOTICS ANONYMOUS

1. We admitted that we were powerless over our addiction, that our lives had become unmanageable.

2. We came to believe that a Power greater than ourselves could restore us to sanity.

3. We made a decision to turn our will and our lives over to the care of God *as we understood Him*.

4. We made a searching and fearless moral inventory of ourselves.

5. We admitted to God, to ourselves, and to another human being the exact nature of our wrongs.

6. We were entirely ready to have God remove all these defects of character.

7. We humbly asked Him to remove our shortcomings.

8. We made a list of all persons we had harmed and became willing to make amends to them all.

9. We made direct amends to such people wherever possible, except when to do so would injure them or others.

10. We continued to take personal inventory and when we were wrong promptly admitted it.

11. We sought through prayer and meditation to improve our conscious contact with God *as we understood Him*, praying only for knowledge of His will for us and the power to carry that out.

12. Having had a spiritual awakening as a result of these steps, we tried to carry this message to addicts, and to practice these principles in all our affairs.

Reprinted by permission of NA World Services, Inc. All rights reserved. The Twelve Steps of NA reprinted for adaptation by permission of AA World Services, Inc.

NA World Services, PO Box 9999, Van Nuys, CA 91409 818-773-9999

www.na.org

C FEELING WORDS

HAPPY
Festive
Relaxed
Calm
Complacent
Satisfied
Serene
Comfortable
Peaceful
Joyous
Ecstatic
Enthusiastic
Inspired
Glad
Pleased
Grateful
Cheerful
Excited
Cheery
Lighthearted
Carefree
Surprised
Optimistic
Spirited
Vivacious
Brisk
Sparkling
Merry
Generous
Hilarious
Exhilarated
Playful
Elated
Jubilant
Thrilled
Restful
Silly

STRESSED
Anxious
Worried

Restless
Uneasy
Worn out
Strung out
Troubled
Impatient

HURT
Injured
Isolated
Offended
Distressed
Disrespected
Pained
Suffering
Afflicted
Worried
Aching
Crushed
Heartbroken
Cold
Upset
Lonely
Despair
Tortured
Pathetic

ANGRY
Contemptuous
Resentful
Irritated
Enraged
Furious
Annoyed
Inflamed
Provoked
Offended
Sullen
Indignant
Irate
Wrathful
Cross

Sulky
Bitter
Frustrated
Grumpy
Boiling
Fuming
Stubborn
Belligerent
Confused
Awkward
Bewildered
Jealous

CALM
Quiet
Centered
Balanced
Accepting
Cool
Restful
Serene
Patient

FEARLESS
Encouraged
Courageous
Confident
Secure
Independent
Reassured
Bold
Brave
Daring
Heroic
Hardy
Determined
Loyal
Proud
Impulsive
Strong
Alive

DOUBTFUL
Unbelieving
Skeptical
Distrustful
Suspicious
Dubious
Uncertain
Questioning
Evasive
Wavering
Hesitant
Perplexed
Indecisive
Hopeless
Powerless
Helpless
Defeated
Pessimistic
Confused

EAGER
Excited
Earnest
Intent
Impatient
Ardent
Avid
Anxious
Enthusiastic
Proud
Restless
Wishful

SAD
Sorrowful
Unhappy
Depressed
Melancholy
Gloomy
Somber
Dismal
Heavyhearted

Quiet
Mournful
Dreadful
Dreary
Flat
Blah
Dull
In the dumps
Sullen
Moody
Sulky
Out of sorts
Low
Discontented
Discouraged
Disappointed
Concerned
Sympathetic
Compassionate
Choked up
Embarrassed
Shameful
Ashamed
Useless
Worthless
Ill at Ease
Weepy
Vacant
Empty

AFRAID
Fearful
Frightened
Timid
Shaky
Apprehensive
Fidgety
Terrified
Panicky
Tragic
Hysterical

Alarmed
Cautious
Shocked
Horrified
Insecure
Impatient
Nervous
Dependent
Anxious
Pressured
Worried
Suspicious
Hesitant
Awed
Dismayed
Scared
Cowardly
Threatened
Appalled
Petrified
Guiltless
Edgy
Uptight
Immobilized
Paralyzed
Tense

LOVED
Admired
Cared for
Cherished
Treasured
Adored
Liked
Worshiped
Fond of
Attached
Enjoyed
Wanted
Needed

"Just as the forest slowly comes back to life after a wildfire, new growth in ourselves after personal devastation is possible with nurturing and patience."

KAY COLBERT

D Affirmations

I no longer feel the need to control others.

I touch others with love and gentleness.

I am learning to express my love.

I treat myself with kindness and patience.

I can give to others with no strings attached.

I can trust all of my thoughts and emotions.

I will make decisions confidently.

I feel great potential for myself.

I am at peace with myself.

I acknowledge my needs.

I can be playful.

I am intelligent.

I affirm my worth and goodness.

I am tactful in my dealings with others.

I open my heart to my inner child.

I allow my Higher Power to enter my life today.

I can face my fears and work to overcome them.

I take full charge of my life today.

I have a new awareness in my life.

I let serenity flow into my life.

I am a responsible person.

I feel happy.

I feel appreciated today.

I respect myself.

I accept my parents and affirm
my independence from them.

I trust in the serenity my
Higher Power provides.

Today, I will put all negativity behind me.

I can meet new opportunities without fear.

I am loved.

Today, I will rejoice in my abilities.

I have many talents.

My Higher Power loves me.

Today, I have confidence.

I look forward to each new day.

I will be who I am.

I am a loving person.

I am not alone.

I am a strong person.

I am a friendly person.

I am a capable person.

Today, I am a new person.

I am in charge of my life.

I am a friend to myself.

I feel positive about my life.

I can make things happen.

I am calm and tranquil.

Resources

1. "Understanding Spiritual Change and its Impact on Outcomes" by the Hazelden Foundation in their October 2009 online newsletter, *The Voice*.

2. "Remembering the Good Times Helps Alcoholics Stay Sober." This summarizes a study by Sarah Davies and Professor Gail Kinman that was presented on April 16, 2010 at the British Psychological Society's Annual Conference.

3. Excellent resources to learn more about mindfulness:

   Full Catastrophe Living by Jon Kabat-Zinn, Delta: 1990.

   Mindfulness-Based Relapse Prevention for Addictive Behaviors by Sarah Bowen, PhD, Neha Chawla PhD, and G. Alan Marlatt PhD, Guilford Press: 2010.

   Mindfulness-Based Cognitive Therapy for Depression by Zindel V. Segal, PhD, J. Mark G. Williams, DPhil, and John D. Teasdale, PhD, Guilford Press: 2012.

   Online: UC San Diego Center for Mindfulness; University of Massachusetts Medical School Center for Mindfulness.

4. *Games for Actors and Non-Actors,* 2nd Ed, by Augusto Boal, Routledge Publishers, 1992

5. "Drumming out Drugs" by Michael Winkelman, PhD, in The American Journal of Public Health, 2003 April (93)4: 647-651. This may be accessed at: www.ncbi. Nih.gov/pmc/articles/pmc/PMC1447805/

Alphabetical Index of Activities

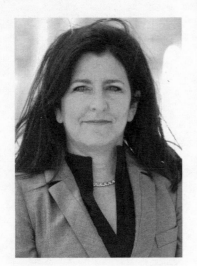

Kay Colbert is a Licensed Clinical Social Worker in private practice. Kay specializes in substance abuse and addictive behaviors, mental health issues, trauma, anxiety, and women's issues. She lectures on mental health, addiction, trauma and mindfulness topics at local and national workshops and conferences. Kay has experience in both private and nonprofit settings. A native of London, England, Kay lives in Dallas, Texas and Whitefish, Montana. She and her husband of thirty-two years have two adult children.

kay@kaycolbert.com   www.kaycolbert.com

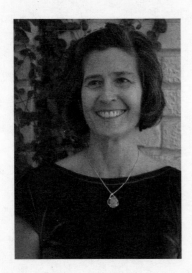

Roxanna Erickson-Klein is a Licensed Professional Counselor and Licensed Chemical Dependency Counselor in private practice. She has experience in pain management and hospice care, substance abuse and addictive behaviors. A Registered Nurse with a Doctorate in Public Administration, she is on the Board of Directors of the Milton H. Erickson Foundation. She is author of numerous professional articles and is a local and international speaker and teacher. A native of Phoenix, Arizona, she lives in Dallas, Texas with her husband of thirty-nine years. Together they have five adult children.

REricksonKlein@gmail.com   www.erickson-klein.org